JOE ZEMAITIS

ATHLETE • COACH • TEACHER

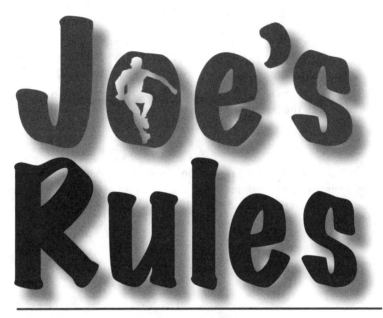

Joe's Rules

**How Every Parent
Can Help Their Child
Excel in Life**
Through Sports

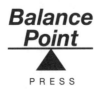

*Balance
Point*

PRESS

Everyone's Talking About...Joe's Rules

"I highly endorse *Joe's Rules* as the parents' handbook for every team and every teacher – athletic, academic, and performing arts. What an amazing change for the better would be accomplished if every parent and coach, volunteer through professional, would read this book and put into practice its principles. I'm encouraging every parent I know to do their children a huge favor by gifting a copy of *Joe's Rules* to every one of their teachers and coaches!"

> *– Nancy Schlueter,*
> *ASCA Level V and USS & NCAA Division I Coach*
> *and Swim technique specialist to many world-class*
> *swimmers and Olympic medalists*

"Joe has nailed it!! There is no better guide book for parents who want to offer their children all the benefits of sports than *Joe's Rules*!"

> *– Pierre Lafontaine*
> *CEO, Swimming Canada*

"*Joe's Rules* is the book every parent should read. In a unique way, Joe combines the energy, optimism and commitment of a 27-year-old with wisdom and experience decades beyond his years – and the result is nothing less than life-changing. *Joe's Rules* has important messages about sports and life that every parent should hear – regardless of the age of their child."

> *– Joy Russell*
> *General Chair, Arizona Swimming, Inc.*

"I am amazed at the insights *Joe's Rules* offers parents in raising their children to be productive, healthy, and ambitious members of our society. As a parent of two of Joe's swimmers and an experienced teacher, I appreciate all that Coach Joe has inspired my children to achieve. Joe's message is a gift for both parent and child."

> *– Kaia Hart*
> *First grade teacher with a Masters in Education*

"One gift a parent can give a child is participation in athletics. I am the person I am today because of swimming. My outlook on life today might be different if I had not been allowed to make swimming my own."

> *– Amy Van Dyken*
> *Six-time Olympic Gold Medalist*

"Coach Joe is an awesome swim coach. He has helped me reach my goals... and set new ones."

> *– Braxton Bilbrey*
> *Set world record at age seven...*
> *youngest to swim Alcatraz*

JOE ZEMAITIS

ATHLETE • COACH • TEACHER

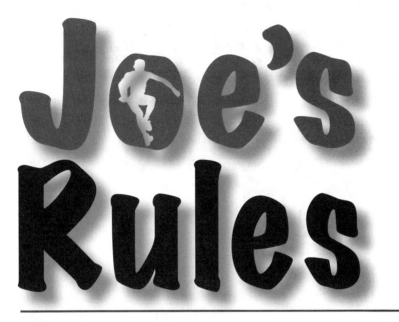

Joe's Rules

How Every Parent
Can Help Their Child
Excel in Life
Through Sports

FOREWORD BY AMY VAN DYKEN
SIX-TIME OLYMPIC GOLD MEDALIST

This publication is designed to provide competent and reliable information re-
garding the subject matter covered. However, it is sold with the understanding
that the author and publisher are not engaged in rendering professional advice.
The authors and publisher specifically disclaim any liability that is incurred from
the use or application of the contents of this book.

If you purchased this book without a cover you should be aware that this book
may have been stolen property and reported as "unsold and destroyed" to the publisher. In such case neither the author nor the publisher has received any payment
for this "stripped book."

Photographs courtesy of The Arizona Republic, John Zemaitis and Robert Oliver

Joe's Rules, Swim Neptune, Team Alcatraz and FAST — The Foundation
for Aquatic Safety and Training are trademarks of Joe Zemaitis

Published by   **Balance
              Point**
              ▲
              PRESS

Visit our Web sites at www.joesrules.com

ISBN-13: 978-0-9795777-0-3
ISBN-10: 0-9795777-0-5

First Edition: June 2007

To Jim Steen

who believed in this book before the first word was written

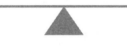

JOE'S RULES

TABLE OF CONTENTS

FOREWORD

In most every child's life there is someone who brings out the very best in them. Someone who sees great things in them …a special stage where they can excel.

I am the person I am today because of swimming and the competition it provided. And my outlook on life today might be very different if I had not been allowed to make swimming my own.

I've known many people who were "supposed" to make the Olympic team, only to fall short at the trials. It's a reminder that no one knows who will make the team, especially the parent of a young child.

When I was growing up, I would hear, "Eat your dinner," "Clean your room," and "Do your homework." Never once did I hear the words, "Train hard and win so you can go to the Olympics." I won my six gold medals through my own persistence…not that of my parents.

Growing up as a severe asthmatic, I was often limited in what activities I could do. I was unable to do many of the things my peers could and, filled with frustration, spent many nights crying to my mom.

Then one summer I found swimming, and fell in love.

I was not the best on the team—not even close. But I was with my friends and would swim a lap when my lungs would allow. My parents were so thrilled that I was outside, doing something I loved (and not having an asthma attack that would inevitably land me in a hospital room for a few days). Swimming must have seemed like a gift to them. Their last thought was to push me to go to practice or to exclaim to the world, "I have a daughter who will be in the Olympics one day." Who would have believed them anyway? And, for that matter, who can ever know with certainty which young athletes will eventually make the team?

One gift that a parent can give a child is the gift of participation in athletics. Another gift they can give is the gift of allowing a child to grow and learn about themselves through a sport. A parent should not take that gift away from a child… and not forget that they had their time as a child, their chance to play the game. Today, the field belongs to their children and their friends.

No one will ever know for sure… but I often wonder if I would have won a gold medal—or even made the team—if I had been chasing someone else's dream. My guess is that I may have ended up being so resentful of my parents and swimming that I may have taken up professional TV-watching, just to spite them. I'll never know for sure because I had great parents who gave me the gift of sports. That gift included learning how to train, compete, win, and even how to lose… all on my own.

Joe's Rules is written by a young man who understands both the drive and passion of a world-class athlete and the universal value of the life lessons of sports. Its messages will impact generations of young people and enrich lives the world over.

– Amy Van Dyken
Six-time Olympic Gold Medalist

ACKNOWLEDGMENTS

It's been my experience that in order to attain success in life, you have to surround yourself with successful people. As I pursued my triathlon career, I was fortunate to have people in my life who went out of their way to help me. And as I set out to develop the best swim team in Arizona, I made sure I surrounded myself with the best; I recruited the best coaching talent available because great coaches can help to inspire great athletes. We continue to learn from each other and work together to create a great team.

My unique perspective on youth sports comes from swimming competitively from age seven through college and ultimately transitioning into the sport of triathlon. My experiences as one of the top amateur triathletes in the U.S. and my successful start to a pro career were aided tremendously by Dominic Arthur, Joseph Coe, Don Giardina, Pierre Lafontaine, Jeff Lockwood, Dr. Alan Palmer, and Rich and Penny Post.

Just as I couldn't develop to the best of my athletic ability by myself or create a top-level competitive swim team by myself, this book would not have been possible without help from a number of different people. It truly was a team effort.

The ideas for this book have been percolating for years. Since I started Swim Neptune in 2002, I found myself constantly explaining my philosophy of sports, coaching, and life—and how it all fits together. A great way to be able to reach and serve the most people with these positive messages about sports was through a book. I strongly believe you can strive and reach the highest levels of sport, which I have been able to do, and have fun along the way. I have spent a lifetime participating in and coaching youth sport. I have participated in some of the top programs in the country and trained alongside of kids who would go on to represent the U.S.A. in the Olympics. Though most young athletes will never reach that level of sport, all benefit from the opportunities that sport provides. True success lies in proportion to the percentage of potential realized.

Two years ago, Jim Steen was the person who explicitly encouraged me to write a book about youth sports, and I sent him each chapter as it was written. This accountability and consistent feedback kept me on track to finish the manuscript; without his help, this book would still be just in my head and not on paper.

It takes a lot of work to turn a bunch of ideas on the written page into the finished product that you see here. Special thanks to the people who took time to read early drafts of the book and provide important insight: Stacey Bilbrey, Leisa Bryan, Kathleen Buckstaff, Don Giardina, Phil Levine, Jeff Lockwood, Heather Logan, Rich Post, and Deborah Westerfield.

Thanks to the people who came into the picture at just the right time to take this book from a manuscript to what you see here. Blair Singer took considerable time from his own writing to help get me started with mine. Several of the concepts I describe in the book originated with Blair's approach to business and sales and are modified to relate to youth sports. Mona Gambetta was the driving force in taking this from a rough manuscript to a finished product. I have never met someone with as much energy and expertise... someone who is so excited to share her knowledge with others. Elizabeth Day offered excellent clarity and insights in refining the message. Kevin Stock designed the cover and layout of the book that is everything I ever could have pictured in my mind's eye. Jen Stern was instrumental in completing the chapter on nutrition and was eager to share her expertise in the field with me. Thanks to Amy Van Dyken-Rouen who wrote the Foreword for the book and who has been so excited to share her passion for swimming and the experience gained at the absolute highest levels of sport with swimmers on Swim Neptune.

Thank you to my parents who allowed sports to play such a large role in my life and who have been supportive through it all. Thanks to my older sister Amy whom I was always chasing in an effort to match her accomplishments in the pool, and my younger brother John whom I had—frantically...and ultimately unsuccessfully—tried to stay ahead of.

I believe that any coach is the product of his previous coaches and his observations of others in the field. Thanks to the multitude of great coaches I have had over the years in different sports who have helped to mold my philosophy. Thanks to all the swimmers I have coached over the years who have provided me the opportunity to refine this philosophy and who have challenged me to challenge them to gain the greatest success in the pool and in life.

INTRODUCTION

It was dawn aboard the *Bravo*, Memorial Day weekend 2002. I was experiencing a "quarter-life crisis" as I watched the sun rising over the Vermillion Sea off the western coast of San Carlos, Mexico.

I had graduated from college two weeks earlier and wasn't sure what the next step should be. Although I had long considered going to law school, I had just spent my last college semester as an intern in Washington, D.C., and the more I saw of the legal profession, the less sure I was that it was the right fit for me.

As I felt the waves gently rock the *Bravo*, I reflected on my life. I knew how to swim before I could walk, and I had wanted to be a scuba diver since I was six years old. Here I was, finally on my first dive trip, getting in four to five dives a day. For as long as I could remember, I had always known what I wanted. I always had a goal and there was always the next step to take. During my freshman year in college, I competed in the Ironman Triathlon in Hawaii and set a world record; at age eighteen, I became the youngest person to finish the race in less than ten hours. What I had thought of as the pinnacle of my athletic career proved only to be the beginning. Following the Ironman, I continued setting goals and enjoyed enough success in the sport to consider making it my profession.

I knew I was passionate about sports, but was unsure about which life path to follow. Do I join the "real world" and get a "real job"? Should I push ahead with law school, even though I was becoming less sure of that with each passing day? Was it the right time to step away from sports and transition into "real life"? What were my options? What was the right choice for me?

I had taken quite a few psychology classes in college and had become fascinated with symbolism. In psychology, water—specifically the ocean—is a symbol of the unconscious because of the intricate world that lies beneath the surface. The analogy was coming alive for me that weekend as I was diving repeatedly into that newfound aquatic wonderland.

Back on the boat between dives, I sorted through my options for the future. I thought about where my passion was. What was my core genius? What could I do better than anyone else? I thought about what I enjoyed the most and when I created the most value for other people. It kept coming back to sports and coaching. Having grown up in the culture of youth sports, I had a very good idea of what worked and what didn't work. I had played a handful of sports for dozens of different coaches, putting in countless hours of training. Then, in my senior year of college, I wrote a 150-page thesis titled, "The Kingdom, the Power, and the Glory: The Meaning of Sport in Modern America."

Was it possible to turn my passions into a career? Standing there aboard the *Bravo*, I decided it was. Not only that, I decided it was possible for me to create a job for myself that would allow me the flexibility to continue to train and race triathlon at the highest level. I spent the rest of the trip outlining my vision for a successful swim team that I would coach. When I got home, I set about putting the pieces in place, including finding a facility with a pool and people who believed in my program. On September 1, 2002, I started my team, Swim Neptune.

In the last four years of coaching and competing, I've found myself explaining my personal philosophies time and again. While on the surface they're about sports, what lies beneath are my core beliefs about personal development and being the best you can be.

In the four years since, I've seen my triathlon hobby transform into a professional career, and I've watched the swim team I started grow beyond anything I could have imagined while on the *Bravo*. I presented an alternative to what was being offered in youth swimming in the Phoenix area and found a huge number of people interested. The team that started at one pool with twenty kids grew into a program that's now at five pools across the Phoenix metro area, with over 250 kids in the year-round competitive and pre-competitive programs.

My personal growth in the sport of triathlon mirrored the phenomenal growth of my swim team. Since 2002, I've competed in six world championship races. I've raced on five continents and in eleven countries—all over North America, South America (Chile), Australia, Asia (Malaysia, Thailand, and Singapore), and Europe (France, Spain, and Denmark). In 2005, I finished fifth at my first Long Course Pro National Championship. Later that year, I raced in the Ironman Triathlon World Championship; as the second youngest pro in a field of eighty-eight entrants, I finished sixty-second overall and seventh out of thirteen Americans.

In the last four years of coaching and competing, I've found myself explaining my personal philosophies time and again. While on the surface they're about sports, what lies beneath are my core beliefs about personal development and being the best you can be. In April 2005, my friend and mentor Blair Singer wrote a piece titled "Joe's Rules" for an e-mail publication, using three of the sayings I often repeat to my swimmers. He used each of these "sporting rules" to illustrate "life's rules." When he told me that he received the most positive feedback he ever had from similar publications, I became even more motivated and inspired to write this book. I realized how many people are genuinely interested in being the best they can be, and even more so in helping their children find their core genius and reach their greatest potential. What follows in the next ten chapters is an exploration of the rules I live by and teach to my students.

CHAPTER ONE

NATURAL TALENT

▲

Joe's Rule #1: "Every child is a genius."

Without exception, every child has a core genius. What does this mean? It means that your child has a natural talent. There's something he or she is particularly good at; there's something your child enjoys and it's likely to be their individual path to success. It's that one thing that sets your child apart and the one thing they can do better than anyone else.

It seems to me that the happiest people are those who have experienced the joy of working within their core genius. On the other hand, the most frustrated people are those who never found their core genius or are ignoring their calling for whatever reason. Your role as a parent is to help your child discover what their core genius is and then support them as they develop it. While your child's core genius may not be a particular sport, having them play sports—either competitive or non-competitive—is a great way to help you and your child discover where their genius lies.

The Moment of Victory

On May 22, 2006, a young swimmer made international news. CNN had live coverage of his swim and, for a couple of hours that day, stories of death, destruction, 26.5 million cases of identity theft, and the projected "critical" hurricane season took a backseat to his story. The next day, he appeared on *Good Morning America* and *CNN's American Morning*. Why? Because that morning,

Braxton Bilbrey, age seven, became the youngest person ever to swim from Alcatraz to San Francisco.

Braxton started swimming with my year-round swim team, Swim Neptune, in August of 2005. He practiced two to three times per week (as recommended for his age) and showed an amazing feel for the water, especially for a kid who had just turned seven. In October of 2005, he asked his parents if he could swim every day, and they in turn asked for my advice. Initially, I was skeptical; in general, I don't think it's a good idea for a seven-year-old to do any sport every day. Pretty soon, however, he showed me, and then the world, that he wasn't your average seven-year-old. What made Braxton different was that he knew exactly what he wanted and he was determined to accomplish his goal.

That last week of May in 2006, Braxton was a rock star. There were five news crews awaiting his arrival at the airport in Phoenix the day after his swim. The next morning when he got to school, there were two news crews waiting to film "Braxton's first day back at school after his record-breaking swim." Braxton was the most popular kid at school that day. He was mobbed on the playground, and then the entire school crowded into the cafeteria for a congratulatory assembly. The school went all out: each class had made a poster congratulating Braxton; they played the Olympic theme as we walked to the podium; and they had an audio/visual presentation of all the media attention he had received in the previous two days.

Before Braxton and I took questions from the kids, I told the excited crowd of students that there were two things I wanted to tell them. First, what they were seeing was equivalent to walking into the last two minutes of a movie. They saw their classmate receive the glory, the acclaim, and media attention that very few of us will ever see in our lifetime. What they didn't see was everything that went into preparing for the swim. While most of them envied him when he was the center of attention, I doubt any of them envied him when there was snow in the Phoenix area in early March. That day, when they were still warm in bed, Braxton was jumping into Lake Pleasant. Conditions that day showed a forty-degree air temperature and a fifty-two-degree water temperature. Braxton was in the water for seventy-five minutes. As I explained to Braxton's peers, no great accomplishment is attained without great sacrifice.

Everyone wants success, but comparatively few want to put in the work required to achieve greatness.

The other important point I wanted the students to understand is that every kid is a genius. Some know what their core genius is, others need direction to help them discover it. That's where coaches, teachers, parents, and mentors come in; it's our job to help children recognize and unlock their core genius.

Braxton tapped into his core genius and was eventually met with media attention and worldwide congratulations. However, even if his name had never been splashed across a newspaper or television, his victory would be no less. His success came not just in the final moment of accomplishment, but in each step of the journey that led to that moment of victory.

The Road to Victory

Braxton's core genius isn't swimming (at least not at this moment). What I told Braxton over and over after his swim was that his accomplishment was never about swimming. It wasn't about setting a world record for the youngest crossing. It wasn't about the interviews or the cameras or the reporters or seeing himself on television. I wasn't proud of him because he won a few minutes of fleeting fame. I was proud of him because he set a goal, put in an enormous amount of hard work to achieve it, and succeeded beyond his own wildest expectations. Braxton's core genius was being able to create a vision and accomplish it without fear. If he transfers that mentality into other areas, he'll be extraordinarily successful in whatever he attempts in life.

Braxton's vision for May 22, 2006 first took form five months earlier. He came to me in January of 2006 with a magazine in his hand and showed me an article about a boy who, at the age of nine, set the record for the youngest crossing from Alcatraz to San Francisco. Braxton wanted to know if I thought he could break the record. I thought he meant that he wanted to do it sometime before he turned nine, meaning he would have a year and a half to train. I was wrong. He wanted to do it as soon as possible. He had already talked to his parents about his idea, and once he convinced them that he was really serious, they told him to talk to his coach.

He came to talk to me about his goal at exactly the right time. With the

> *Braxton's core genius was being able to create a vision and accomplish it without fear.*

beginning of the new year, I had taken stock of what was important to me. So much of my life had been about pursuing my own goals. Along the way, certain people had come into my life at exactly the right moments to help me achieve those goals. I was starting to feel that it was time to repay the people who had gotten me to where I was.

For years, Dominic Arthur, a former professional triathlete in Phoenix, helped me train for triathlon and gave me equipment I could have never afforded on my own. In all that time, he never asked me for anything. Then one day, he told me how I could pay him back: When I was a successful professional athlete, I was to help someone else in the same way he helped me. I had always wondered how I would find someone with the same sort of impossible goals I had when I was a kid. Little did I know that he would find me.

I talked to Braxton's parents and we mapped out a plan to help Braxton reach his goals. When the previous record holder, a nine-year-old, completed his swim, he used the opportunity to raise money for victims of Hurricane Katrina. When I suggested to Braxton that he use his swim to raise money for a good cause, he said, "To stop kids from dying in pools." The reason Braxton learned to swim when he was three years old was so that he would be safe around water. Braxton's parents had long stressed the importance of pool safety and drilled into him what it takes to be safe around water. Since 2000, over 130 kids under the age of five drowned in the Phoenix area. Most of these drownings involved unsupervised children around swimming pools, or kids who somehow managed to slip outside and get around a pool fence. Now we had a dual mission: set the record for the youngest crossing and raise money and awareness for drowning prevention programs in Arizona.

In order to begin, we would have to get Braxton a wetsuit and he would have to try it out in the pool. Then we would go to a lake around Phoenix while the water was still bitterly cold and see how he'd do swimming in open water.

Braxton was a strong swimmer in a pool, but when you add limited visibility, frigid waters, choppy conditions, and the creeping thought of what could be lurking in the dark depths, the obstacles and challenges multiply.

Braxton passed every test with flying colors. Each time he practiced in open water, it was better than the time before. He continued swimming in the pool four times a week for two hours a day, and we took five weekend trips to open water for swims between one and two hours.

How hard is too hard to push this kid?

As a coach I was in a difficult situation. I had to know what Braxton's breaking point was. I needed to know how far he could go because if we went past that point during the Alcatraz swim, we would need to pull him out of the water. He had to know what it felt like to get out of his comfort zone—but still, he was only seven. How far should you push a seven-year-old? As a parent, how far should you push your child at any age? The answer will always depend on the child's personality and their level of motivation.

The desire to swim Alcatraz had to come exclusively from Braxton himself. Because he wanted to swim Alcatraz more than anything else, he didn't get burned out swimming up to ten hours a week and logging up to fifteen miles a week in the water. I have parents come to me, concerned their seven-year-old is burned out when they swim twice a week for forty-five minutes. That demonstrates how important desire and goals are. You take one seven-year-old with an "impossible goal" and he'll swim ten hours a week and come back for more. Take another seven-year-old without a goal or strong desire related to swimming, and an hour and a half a week in the pool leads to perceived burnout. Success becomes more attainable when you're doing something you want to be doing.

Braxton's success had very little to do with swimming. His genius was the ability to come up with a goal on his own and, most importantly, stick with it even when it was difficult. Sure there were days when he was tired or sore or felt overwhelmed. The training schedule would have knocked out most adults. Very few people of any age have the ability to create such goals, and fewer still have the courage to accomplish them fearlessly.

The Fearless Pursuit of a Goal

In April, Braxton's parents went to San Francisco to tour Alcatraz and give Braxton an idea of what he was up against. The first thing he said when he saw Alcatraz Island from San Francisco was, "Oh, that's not that far." There was never any fear. He fended off every question about sharks (that every interviewer asked about), shrugging it off saying that he would just "punch the shark in the nose." Working with Braxton every day, I learned about my own tendency to over-think situations and let reasons why I "can't" do something creep into my mind.

When the day of the Alcatraz swim arrived, Braxton was still as fearless as ever. We took a boat out to the island early in the morning, and by the time we arrived, he was freezing. The wind created by the boat skimming out toward Alcatraz chilled us from head to toe. The last thing I told him before we jumped into the fifty-six-degree water was that it was just another swim. I told him to forget all the cameras and people asking him questions, to just swim "right on my feet" (directly behind me, staying as close as possible) like we had done repeatedly over the previous four months. With that, we jumped in the water, swam over to Alcatraz, put our feet on dry land, then pushed off toward the San Francisco skyline.

It wasn't until about ten minutes into the swim that I first picked my head up to ask how he was doing. He had warmed up, found a rhythm, and was ready to go. I only stopped once more to check up on him because he wanted to just keep going. We had trained to just complete it, not to finish so quickly! Braxton made the official crossing in forty-seven minutes and we were besieged by reporters at the beach. He had accomplished his goal: He broke the record.

Setting Goals

Even if a goal ends up unattained, it's a not a failure; it's a learning experience. If you fail to accomplish a goal, you didn't lose anything. If Braxton had been unable to complete the swim, the journey would still have been a success. He didn't have a world record when he started the quest, and if he hadn't completed it, he wouldn't have been worse off than when he started. If he was unable to complete the crossing, a learning experience on goal-setting may have turned into a learning experience on perseverance—as I have no doubt he would have trained more and succeeded on a second attempt.

An inevitable question after an accomplishment like this is: "What next?" On the beach right after the swim, he proclaimed on national TV that he wanted to swim the English Channel (first time I heard about it) or the Swim Around the Rock, a three-and-a-half-mile swim from San Francisco around Alcatraz and back. It was a question I didn't like because this was never about "what next." When reporters asked me that question, I told them, "He's going back to being seven again." This was never about getting massive media attention, it was never about trying to outdo himself every year or make headlines in the process. It was about a kid with a goal and his story of how hard he worked to achieve it. If he sets a new goal, I'll do what I can to help him get there. However, if it's not coming from him, if it's only "his" goal because he feels like he's *obligated* to do it, he won't have the same success. For a goal to be *successfully* attained, you have to be true to yourself and pursue it for the right reasons.

Pre-Paving the Road to Victory

A major ingredient for success is setting yourself up for the opportunity when it arrives. Braxton was able to achieve his goal because of his early dedication to swimming before the goal even crossed his mind. If he had been swimming for only an hour a day, twice a week, he wouldn't have been in the position to achieve his goal once he was inspired by the magazine article. Because he had been working hard, showing tremendous determination and dedication, reading about the record-breaking swim ignited something in him and he was ready to step up and take the challenge. Because his confidence had been building during months of hard work, he *knew inside himself* that he could do the swim from Alcatraz, even if he wasn't fully aware of what the challenge would require when he first read the article. It all begins with believing in yourself. Once you believe in yourself, you start to act in ways that support that belief and encourage it even further.

When I was twelve years old, I wrote a goal on the ceiling above my bed reminding me that I was going to do the Ironman at the age of eighteen. Two things on the wall in Braxton's room struck me when I was at his house doing a series of radio interviews after the swim. The first was a poster of Michael Phelps with the following quote: "Some kids worship heroes. Others become them." The second was a picture of the Arizona Diamondbacks home ballpark with the words "Braxton Bilbrey MVP" superimposed over a generic scoreboard, a remnant of picture day from a Little League baseball season.

Today, Braxton has his Michael Phelps poster signed by Phelps himself. Braxton also has a framed picture of the day in June 2006 when he threw out the first pitch at a Diamondbacks game and his name is on the scoreboard for real. It gave me chills when I thought about it. It didn't happen by accident. Braxton was a motivated, goal-oriented kid long before he could even understand what those words meant. His dedication and vision paid huge dividends; when the opportunity to have a chance at greatness came calling, he was prepared.

Unlocking the Core Genius

Braxton was lucky to have his core genius emerge so early in his life, but he's hardly alone. Braxton is the face of millions of kids who have a genius. He represents *all* kids because all kids have a superstar inside. For all that Braxton accomplished, he's not that gifted or that unusual. He's a normal eight-year-old who lets his room get messy, has trouble tying his shoes, and fights with his three-year-old brother. The difference is that he found his core genius and accomplished something that the world noticed. The genius in him emerged. Early on, his parents gave him the freedom to try all sorts of different sports. He was always miles ahead of his peers in about every sport he tried. But it wasn't about the sports at all. His talent wasn't just as an athlete. His talent was that he was far ahead of kids twice his age in mental strength and determination.

In order to accomplish something great, a child needs three things: a natural talent, the motivation and dedication to use that talent, and a great support crew behind them. That means they need their parents to be supportive without being overbearing, parents who won't let them give up at the first sign of adversity.

Having a core genius is far from unique; it's there inside everyone. Parents can help kids identify their individual greatness and let that part of them shine. How? By noticing what they're good at and what comes naturally to them. Notice what they enjoy doing and what motivates and inspires them. The more we allow children to explore different paths and expose them to different things, the more likely they are to discover their true core genius.

I've discovered along the way that helping someone with *their* goals can help unleash *your* productive power in your own life. By coaching a team of hundreds of great kids, by writing a book in order to reach more people with a life-changing message of success, and by working with one particular kid on his own goals, *I've learned a lot and grown in the process.* As you help to unlock and unleash the core genius in your child, I encourage you to keep an eye open to see how you can use the experience to further fulfillment in your own life.

Chapter Summary

Every parent wants their child to be successful. Braxton Bilbrey's story illustrates what steps you can take with your child to help lead them to *their own* moments of victory. It begins with exposing your child to a variety of experiences so that you can help them identify their core genius. As you'll see in the following chapters, participation in sports is an ideal way to help your child see where their true talent lies (whether it's on the field or off the field). Once you identify the core genius, it's important to set goals with your child. Goals, when rooted in a child's core genius, pave the road to success.

CHAPTER TWO

THE SPORT DEPENDS ON THE CHILD

Joe's Rule #2: "Every child must play sports."

It's often said, "Sports aren't for everyone." I completely disagree. Certain sports aren't right for everyone, but all children have to be active. Before deciding which sport your child should be playing, you have to first take a good look at your child's personality. That will help you recognize how your child, in particular, can benefit from sports. You need to begin with the end in mind by answering the following question: "To what end?" It's critical to know *why* you want your child playing sports. What do you want them to get out of it? What do they hope to get out of the experience? By first considering "who" your child is and "why" they must play sports, you'll have meaningful direction when choosing the "what"—the perfect sport and program for your child. So, let's begin by looking at "who" today's children are.

Today's Children

As a parent, you didn't have to participate in organized sports and you turned out just fine—right? I agree, but today's world and today's children are different. You didn't have to join a soccer team to be active. You walked to school (uphill both ways in snow up to your chest, right!?) and then had PE— a real PE class! When you got home after school, you played outside until dinnertime. You lived in a world where you could go to the park by yourself. You could ride your bike around the neighborhood and come home for dinner when

Certain sports aren't right for everyone, but all children have to be active.

the streetlights came on. You didn't spend your time after school sitting in front of the TV or playing video games; you only had three channels, and let's face it—you could only play Pong for so long. You were active, you were healthy, and you didn't need adults organizing your games for you.

So much for the good old days! Today, it might even be considered child neglect if you let your kids go to the park unsupervised. You wouldn't dream of letting your kids "hang out" all over the neighborhood for hours on end. And while your parents could count on the schools to provide serious PE, it isn't the current reality. Only one state (Illinois) has required daily PE for kindergarten through twelfth grade. Many schools have only a twenty-minute period for PE. That's a start, but not nearly the sixty minutes of activity a day, minimum, that the Surgeon General recommends. In the days of budget cuts and standardized tests, PE is among the first to go. Even when children do have PE, there doesn't seem to be a lot of activity going on. A study by John Cawley of Cornell University shows that high school students are active for an average of sixteen minutes per PE class. Another study done in a county of Texas shows that the children in elementary school are active for only 3.4 minutes per PE period.

Some parents decide to take matters into their own hands. It's possible for parents to provide their children with fitness opportunities, but not ideal. Unless you can make a serious family commitment to an hour after school every day, it's usually not realistic or practical. And please don't bring your child to the gym and make them walk on the treadmill for an hour. Exercise at that age should be fun and exciting; they should be learning new skills and exploring the strengths and limitations of their changing bodies. Ideally, the physical activity will also provide great interaction with other kids. Walking on a treadmill is a task of drudgery and won't inspire a lifetime love of fitness.

Most adults recognize the need for their children to be active and realize that they can't count on schools to provide a fitness outlet. The majority of parents also readily admit that signing their child up for a sports program is more likely to guarantee opportunity for exercise than if they tried to plan and maintain a workout regimen themselves. So then, the question becomes: Which sport is right for my child? Well, that answer depends on who your child is.

Knowing Your Child

Each child is different. If all children were the same, had the same gifts, and were motivated by the same thing, a book about kids and sports would only need to be a single page long. There are lots of different youth sports programs at all levels, and there's certainly one out there that's a great fit for your child. In order to find the perfect program, you need to get a good read on what makes your child tick.

When evaluating your child, try to go beyond sports and see how they approach other parts of life. Are they the student who gets hysterical over a "B" on a report card, or the one who couldn't care less about a "D"? Are they the type who learns a new activity by plunging in headfirst, or by hanging back to see how it's done? Do they get nervous about an upcoming test, or do they tend not to get nervous enough?

By honestly examining where they fall on the spectrum of the three following categories, you'll have a better idea of what motivates them and you'll begin to see how they could benefit from participating in sports. Recognize that wherever a child falls on the range isn't good or bad, it just is what it is. Just as kids have different learning styles in school, they have different athletic personalities that emerge through sports.

Spectrum I: *Laid-Back to Intense*
Simply put, a child who's too laid-back doesn't care enough about something important. A child who's too intense cares way too much about something that's unimportant.

The most laid-back, eight-year-old swimmer I ever coached raced herself to a third place finish in the League Championships. After she completed the race, she was told that she'd been disqualified for a one-hand touch on the breaststroke. This would bring tears from just about every other kid, but not her. She replied, "That's OK. It means somebody else will get to win a medal." Though I hoped that after a season of preparation, the League finals would mean a little bit more than that, I couldn't help but admire an eight-year-old with that kind of perspective.

Intense kids are a different story. They often put incredible pressure on themselves, thus preventing them from performing at optimal levels. The most intense kid I ever knew put pressure on himself to win every race, no matter what it took. He wanted to win (by his own definition) every practice, and in always trying to race sometimes lost sight of the point of practice (which is to improve, not necessarily to compete). He approached school the same way, always wanting the top grade in every class and feeling crushed any time his performance fell short of his high expectations. He couldn't even stand losing at cards!

That was me eighteen years ago. With time, I mellowed out a bit and gained some much needed perspective. It was a long process whereby I gradually realized that most of the things I worried about didn't mean as much as I thought they did. It just takes some people a while to develop the maturity to recognize that. I still have a very intense personality, but I can turn it on and off depending on the situation, recognizing when it matters in the pursuit of my goals.

Chances are your child is somewhere between the two extremes. Maybe they exhibit different behaviors on different days or during different activities. If you watch long enough and carefully enough, you'll see patterns emerge. Once you recognize where your child is on the spectrum, you'll become aware of their needs and their athletic personalities.

One summer, I had two very fast swimmers, both nine-year-old boys, who were at opposite ends of the spectrum. Before the big race, I said to one: "OK, this is it, this is what you've been training for all year. This is your one chance to show everyone how hard you worked. I need you to get up on the blocks and swim the best race of your life." I then went two lanes over to tell the other one: "This is just another meet. I need you to race like you know you can, like we do every day in practice. Just relax and let your best race come out of you." By knowing whether your child tends to be more intense or more laid-back, you can determine how to best support them and how to make playing sports a positive growth experience.

Spectrum II: *Nervous to Confident*

The too-nervous athletes will make themselves physically sick before a game. They'll worry about everything that could go wrong and create a self-fulfilling prophecy of failure. They'll think up excuses in advance in case of failure: "My stomach hurts, I have a headache, and my shoes are too small." They'll repeat them enough so that they become true in their own mind. The confident athlete, on the other hand, will relish competition. They want to be the one to take the shot with the game on the line. They're hoping that the bases will be loaded with the tying run on third when they come to the plate.

Again, most athletes fall somewhere in the middle of the two extremes. Kids who tend to be more confident have an innate trust in their own abilities and live for the opportunity to perform on the athletic stage. For kids who tend to be nervous, playing sports provides the ideal opportunity for them to overcome their fears and learn how to control their nerves. The nervous athlete finally competes enough times and realizes that no matter what happens, life goes on. Getting sick over an impending game isn't going to do any good. This is obviously a critical life lesson that will serve them for the rest of their life.

The nervous athlete is also likely to discover that, with experience, nervousness eventually gives way to confidence. They'll learn not to shy away from a challenge they're prepared to meet simply because they're afraid of it. I had a mother tell me about her eleven-year-old who was nervous about his first week at a new school. He said, "I just can't do it. I can't go. I'm going to throw up." The mother replied, "Then I can stop the car to give you a chance to throw up, but then we're going to keep driving to school."

Spectrum III: *Thinker to Doer*

On one end of this spectrum is the child who says, "Ready. Fire. Aim!" On the opposite end is the one who says, "Ready. Aim. Aim. Aim...."

A mother was telling me about taking her two boys surfing and summed up the difference between them: "The five-year-old just stands up and does it. The seven-year-old thinks about it and misses the wave." The doer doesn't have the patience to wait around. He wants action, he wants speed, he wants to plunge right in and give it a try. The thinker can't bring himself to plunge in. He needs time to go over it in his mind until he's comfortable with the activity. The doer often learns best by experience. The thinker learns from hearing how to do it, from watching someone do it, and finally by trying it himself.

These personalities suit themselves to different sports and different disciplines within a sport. Lance Armstrong talks about how early in his career he just wanted to race. He didn't want to think through the strategy, he just wanted to get on his bike and ride it as fast as he could. He was often in the lead early in the race, only to be caught later by a rider who rode a smarter race. Cycling is described as a "chess game on wheels"; so much of the sport relies on team tactics. Someone who's on their own riding as hard as he can right from the start doesn't stand much of a chance. In the Ironman Triathlon, anyone without specific training and a clear concept

Giving a child complete control over their free time makes about as much sense as giving them complete control over their diet. Kids can't be expected to make the right choices all the time.

of their pace wouldn't make it through the 2.4-mile swim, 112-mile bike and 26.2-mile run.

Certain activities are much better suited to the doer. Some sports require a developed instinct and if you hesitate a split second to think about it, you've already lost. In swimming or track, a split-second delay on the start can be an insurmountable deficit. In baseball, a hitter doesn't have much time to decide whether they want to swing at a particular pitch, and a fielder doesn't have time to think about how they want to play a certain ball. It has to be automatic, done without thinking. I have the "thinker" personality, but when I look back at some of my best races, I don't remember much of them. I was finally able to turn my brain off and just do what I had trained to do.

Of the three different spectrums, this is probably the one where you'll see the least movement. It's very difficult to get a doer to take the time to think through what they're trying to accomplish. It just goes against their nature. They want to get in there and have at it. In a similar way, it's very difficult for the thinker to turn off their brain and just do it. This is the category where the optimum performance will be found in a hybrid model between the two. You want to be a thinker before the game and develop a strategy for success. Once the event starts, a successful athlete needs the ability to trust their training and instincts—and just go for it.

You may have a good idea of where your child falls on each of the three personality spectrums, but there was probably one in particular where you said, "Yep, that's my child!" Once you've taken the time to determine what personality your child exhibits in the three spectrums, their specific needs and how they operate become more obvious. Now that you've answered the "who" question, it's time to answer the "why."

How Can Playing Sports Benefit Your Child?

It's important to find out why your child wants (or doesn't want) to play sports, and it's just as critical for you to have *your* reasons why they should play. Why do you want your child to participate in sports? Wait, did I just commit the sin of sports parenting? Is it wrong to consider your desires when choosing a sport for your kid? Absolutely not. Giving a child complete control over their free time makes about as much sense as giving them complete control over their diet. Kids can't be expected to make the right choices all the time. If you let your child choose what they ate all the time, what would the result be? Would some kids naturally choose a balanced diet? Probably, but most wouldn't. If you gave your child complete control over their free time, would some choose to be active and pursue a healthy lifestyle? Again, some would. Most wouldn't, though.

Remember: Motion can change emotion.

Once you figure out why you want your child in sports, you'll have all the information you need for the next step—helping your child decide which sport to pursue. Until you know the "who" and the "why," you won't know the "what." As you read the following ten reasons why children play sports, keep in mind the personality of your child. Which of the following benefits could your child use?

Ten Reasons Why Children Play Sports

1. *Emotional and Mental Well-Being*

   At all times, the body has four states of being: a mental state, an emotional state, a physical state, and a spiritual state that encompasses the other three states. If you're mentally stressed, emotionally depressed, and physically exhausted, you're obviously in a negative state. When you're feeling "down," it's usually in all three areas at the same time. You don't often feel mentally stressed when you're feeling joyful emotions and physically energetic.

   When you change one of these states, you change them all, and the easiest state to change is the physical. If you're stressed, depressed, and exhausted, and you go work out for twenty minutes, your energy level rises. With that resurgence in energy, your mental and emotional states become more positive. Being active is the best way to improve your mental and emotional states.

Kids are sedentary all day in school. If they spend the rest of their time in front of a TV or computer, they don't have the physical release they need to function at their best. Kids need the shift in the physical state in order to have a positive effect on their mental and emotional well-being. Remember: Motion can change emotion.

2. *Lessons from Your Own Regrets*

Oh no, we're talking about you again. Is this wrong? No, it's an honest answer to why some parents have their kids in a certain activity. Maybe you wish you had these opportunities when you were younger and you want your child to have them. This is surely an admirable reason. I got started in swimming at a young age because my mom didn't put her face underwater until she was twelve. She grew up in Chicago and had no opportunity (or reason) to learn to swim. When she was nine, her family moved to California—the land of swimming pools—and she was scared to death. She missed out on a lot of fun activities because she couldn't go swimming with her friends since she didn't know how. She passed a swimming test in high school, but it was a traumatic experience that she still hasn't forgotten.

My mother was determined to have her children learn to swim at a young age so we wouldn't share her fear of the water. By the age of six months,

Part of being a good parent is helping your child avoid making the same mistakes you made.

each of us three kids was taking the "Mom & Baby" swim lessons and we all developed an early love of the water. That's why I knew how to swim before I could walk.

Maybe you quit a sport or gave up an activity only to realize later how beneficial it would have been if you had stuck with it. Part of being a good parent is helping your child avoid making the same mistakes you made. Learning from personal mistakes is a big part of growing up. There are some mistakes your children will have to learn for themselves, but this isn't one of them. Don't wait until your child is seriously overweight and under-motivated to try to get them interested in a healthy lifestyle. Start young!

3. *Keeping Them Busy*

Like my mom said, "Idle hands are the devil's tools." Soon after we were born, my mom asked her aunt the secret to raising three good kids. The response was, "Keeping them busy." Her aunt's kids were all involved in swimming, activities at church, and/or part-time jobs. Because they were involved in productive activities, they didn't have time to get themselves into trouble.

Signing your child up for sports is far from having your child babysat. Kids aren't just killing time, they're learning skills and lessons that will serve them well for life.

I had two very talented young swimmers on my swim team. Though people came up to their mother and said, "Wow, you must be planning on them going to the Olympics," she confided to me that she'd be happy if all they got out of swimming was learning how to spend their time productively. "As long as they aren't spending all of high school hanging out at the mall, I'll be happy." That's a great attitude. Some kids will go on to great things, even commercial success as athletes, but they're the exceptions. If kids are striving toward their goals as an athlete and not wasting time loitering at the mall every day, they're going to come out ahead—even if they don't end up with a big shoe endorsement deal.

4. *Fitness for Life*

    This is a big one. Whether or not your child exhibits a natural talent in any sport, participation will ensure that they receive the benefits of fitness. Children are becoming overweight earlier and childhood obesity is becoming more and more prevalent. This isn't about vanity. It isn't about looking a certain way or fitting into a certain size. If they're overweight as children, they're setting themselves up for a lifetime of health problems.

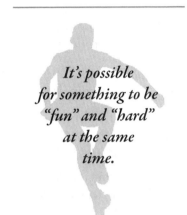

It's possible for something to be "fun" and "hard" at the same time.

Studies show that an obese or overweight child is more likely to grow into an obese or overweight adult and inherit the health and lifestyle problems that go with it.

Finding the middle ground, the healthy middle, is the best road to fitness and a healthy lifestyle. The opposite of a flood—a drought—can be just as deadly. Eating disorders are equally as unhealthy as obesity. You don't want to give your child a complex; you just want them to be healthy.

Sports don't have to be the driving force of your child's life. Maybe your child just isn't an athlete...that's OK. Not everyone is cut out to be a competitive athlete, just as everyone isn't cut out to be an artist. Your child doesn't have to be on a competitive, traveling basketball team to get the benefits of fitness; maybe you just enroll them in the YMCA basketball program. If your child doesn't enjoy sports or isn't particularly good at anything, you just have to look harder. There are many opportunities these days for youth sports beyond the traditional ones like soccer, baseball, and basketball. You just have to look a little deeper and find a sport your child will enjoy doing, one that will keep them active. They'll thank you later.

5. *Fun and Friends*

Nearly all of my friends, with whom I still keep in touch, came from my participation in sports. There's something special about the bond that forms over shared competition. Not only do you have an interest in common, you also have a similar level of commitment if you're in the same program or on the same team. Deciding to enroll your child in sports to help them form friendships is another great reason. It's a forum for kids to interact with each other in a less restrictive way than school. Sports bring together kids of similar ages and interests and give your child the opportunity to be more social.

Not only do kids need to be social, they also need to have fun—and fun is an integral part of any successful program. Kids won't be interested in a program unless it grants them some form of fun. Fun doesn't mean playing games and messing around all the time. It's "fun" for many kids to work extremely hard during the year and watch it pay off in a big way. These are the years when it's important to tie fun and fitness together. As an adult, when you find a great exercise program, you'll notice that it's fun for you. The same is true for kids. If they find a program that meets their needs, it's going to be fun. It's possible to be "fun" and "hard" at the same time.

> *"Fun" means different things to different people; discover what it means to your child.*

After spending the entire day inside at school, kids need a chance to be outside and just be a kid. Since the days of wandering through the neighborhood and running unsupervised at the park are over, you need to pick an activity for them (or with them). If you and your child rank fun as the top priority, look for the program they'll get the most enjoyment out of, even if it's not the one where they'll learn the most or win the most games. You can judge the success of the season based on if they had fun. For me, nothing is more fun than going to a race and competing with the best. I rank that kind of fun far above playing a game. "Fun" means different things to different people; discover what it means to your child.

6. *Being Part of a Team*
   Teams give an individual a chance to participate in something larger than themselves. "Team" is a big buzzword in business and school these days. You form sales teams, research and development teams, and study teams. Learning to be an effective team member is an acquired skill, just like anything else.

> *There's nothing inherently negative about competition; it becomes a problem when sight of all else is lost in a single-minded pursuit of "win at all costs."*

That which is good for the team sometimes has to come first. Learning to put the needs of a team above your own needs is a great life lesson. Kids need to learn to be accountable and realize that their actions affect the well-being of other people. If you're responsible for writing up a section of a team report, and you didn't do it because other things took priority, you're letting down the team. It's not fair to everyone else who put in the work required. Teamwork is necessary not only in the business world and school, but also in every family. Children need to learn that being part of a team (including their family) means cooperation and sacrifice.

Effective teams are able to push each other. You're often able to get more out of yourself as part of a team than you ever would as an individual. It means learning that you show up to practice even if you don't feel your best or you're tired—because the team will suffer in your absence. It means you're there for each other. The earlier a child learns the requirements and value of being part of a team, the better prepared they'll be for all the "teams" they'll eventually be a part of. In addition, if and when they create their own team, no matter what kind of team it is, they'll understand the necessary components for one that's successful.

7. *Independence*

    On the flipside, when kids are part of a team, they also learn a lot about independence. Sports provide kids an opportunity to assert independence and do something for themselves. It can be a great lesson on responsibility because in sports there's always the defining moment when nobody else can do it for you. Whether it's lining up for an important free throw, having to make a split-second pass, or lining up for a big race, nobody else can do it for you.

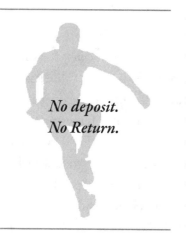

No deposit.
No Return.

By being part of a team, a child learns about the individual roles that each person on the team must play. To win a soccer game, you have to score more goals than the other team; it's as simple as that. But not everyone on the team is trying to score a goal; the goalkeeper, defense, and offense all have to do their jobs in order for the team to win. By giving your child the opportunity to play sports, you're allowing them the chance to assert independence and to take ownership of something.

8. *Competition*

    In today's "everybody wins" mentality, competition gets a bad rap. One reason to enroll your child in sports is so that they're exposed to competition. "Competition" literally means "to strive together." There's nothing inherently negative about competition; it becomes a problem when sight of all else is lost in a single-minded pursuit of "win at all costs."

The world is a competitive place and that isn't going to change. You have to compete with classmates to get good grades, you have to compete with other seniors for slots at a desired college or scholarship opportunities. You have to compete with other applicants for a job and other people for a promotion. Competition is healthy; it encourages and motivates us to do our best. If you're looking to sports to provide an introduction to competition for your child, find a program that promotes the view of competition that you believe in.

Competition in sports helped me to learn how to lose. It's certainly not as much fun as winning! But what I learned personally from sports competition is that I could be happy with a 100 percent effort from myself. I didn't mind losing as long as I could walk away from the competition knowing that I had given 100 percent of what I had that day. Sports can be a great way to teach your child to win with grace and lose with class. Learning how to compete and how to handle competition is part of growing up.

9. *Discipline and Self-Confidence*
Having your child play sports provides an excellent opportunity to teach that little pearl of wisdom

When they don't feel like getting out of bed and going to practice, but they do anyway, they end up feeling good about themselves. The better they feel about themselves, the more self-confidence they have. Not the pseudo-confidence that results from everyone saying how great you are, but the kind of self-confidence that can only be earned, not given.

found on the old Coke bottle: No deposit. No Return. If the work isn't done in practice, then the desired results won't happen because success doesn't come by accident. What you give, you get back.

The discipline required to be successful in sports is the same type of discipline that every child needs to be successful in life. Sports can help develop good habits like giving a full effort, playing by the rules, and being responsible to the coach and to the team. The more a child learns and practices discipline, the better they feel about themselves. It's that simple. All of us, no matter what age we are, feel good when we work hard and especially when we put in the necessary effort even when we don't feel like doing it.

Every time your child goes to practice, completes a drill, or puts any effort toward a goal, they're learning discipline and experiencing the results. When they don't feel like getting out of bed and going to practice, but they do anyway, they end up feeling good about themselves. The better they feel about themselves, the more self-confidence they have. Not the pseudo-confidence that results from everyone saying how great you are, but the kind of self-confidence that can only be earned, not given. This confidence will carry over into the rest of their life. Now they know that a difficult challenge can be tackled and conquered. They know what they're made of.

10. *Athletic Goals: Elite / Collegiate / Professional*

Is it wrong to want your kid to grow up to be a professional baseball player? I say it's no better or worse than if you wanted them to grow up to be a doctor or any other professional. Ultimately, though, children have to want it for themselves. There's a lot of work that goes into being a professional athlete. It's very difficult, if not impossible, to put in the work required when the passion isn't the child's, but belongs to the parent.

A college scholarship is a great goal to strive toward. With the tens of thousands of dollars that my parents invested in our swimming over the years, it's great that it paid off for my brother and sister in the form of nearly full scholarships to Division I schools. But even if there hadn't been a financial windfall at the end of the high school swimming career, my parents certainly wouldn't have looked at that money as wasted.

If a young athlete loves a sport and wants to put it above everything else, it's important to encourage them in their passionate pursuit of excellence. However, you need to think long-term as well. No eight-year-old ever made the Olympics or signed an NFL contract. Doing too much too soon can hurt the future development of an athlete, especially since you won't know until after puberty what their adult body will look like.

Above all else, avoid putting unrealistic expectations on your child. It's fine to secretly hope that they'll one day be the Olympic champion. It's also fine to hope your child grows up to be the Surgeon General. Just stay away from the day-to-day coaching and heaping mounds of pressure to succeed when they aren't ready to handle it. You wouldn't go on daily diatribes about homework and ride your fourth-grader, telling them, "This A- on your spelling test yesterday isn't acceptable if you want to get into a good high school, then a good college, then a good medical school, then a good residency and internship, then make the political connections necessary to get yourself appointed Surgeon General." You can see how ridiculous it sounds in that context. Be careful not to make a similar mistake with sports.

Helping Your Child Decide Which Sport to Play

We've just covered many different reasons for having your child play sports and chances are, certain benefits just jumped off the page at you. You may want your child involved in sports for all of the reasons mentioned, or you may be saying to yourself, "If nothing else, I hope they can get 'this' out of the whole youth sports experience." What you decide will have major implications on the sport and program that you select with your child. If you want your child to have fun more than anything else, then the program you select will be very different from the one chosen by the parent who harbors professional aspirations for their budding superstar. Be clear about why your child wants to play sports and why you want them to play sports. Talk to your child about what you hope they'll get out of the experience and what they hope to get out of it.

Chapter Summary

You have to begin with the end in mind, focusing on the question, "To what end?" I've seen many athletes, parents, and coaches unhappy with their sport. In many cases, they lost sight of why they were involved. Until you can answer the "why" question, you can't move forward meaningfully. What makes your child tick? What do you want your child to get out of sports? What do they want to get out of sports? These questions are crucial to deciding the next step—what type of sports program would most benefit your child. Whatever the choice, *be supportive.*

CHAPTER THREE

KNOW YOUR OPTIONS

Joe's Rule #3: "Know your child and find the right fit."

Finding the right program begins with finding the right sport for your child. There are sports that get you in shape and sports you have to get in shape for. Some sports require fine motor skills, some gross motor skills. Some require concentration, others endurance. Some are individual sports and some are team sports. Different characteristics can be gained and developed by different sports.

Based on your child's personality, body type, and motivation, they'll be attracted to different sports. There are always exceptions to every rule, but use common sense when helping them choose a sport. If they need to be active and constantly running around, then baseball probably wouldn't be a good choice for them. If they're the smallest kid in their class, playing basketball might not be the ideal choice. If they're the tallest in their class, pursuing gymnastics might be setting them up for failure. When I was growing up, my dad made football completely off limits. He'd seen too many kids who got seriously injured playing football. He wouldn't even let me play flag football: "Because you'll be good at it and want to play tackle." You have to use common sense and your best judgment as a parent, but with that said, if the child shows an interest in trying a sport, then let them go for it. Encourage them to explore their passions.

With very few exceptions, there are no "right" or "wrong" programs. At the same time, not every program is right for everyone. When choosing the

> *If the child shows an interest in trying a sport, then let them go for it.*

program for your child, you'll first need to consider the appropriate level. Once you decide on the level, it's time to choose a program that's aligned with your expectations, goals, and vision for your child. Then, as your child grows and changes, you need to be aware of their developmental stages so that the programs you choose continue to be an appropriate fit. And finally, along the way, you'll need to know when it's time to move up to the next level and when it's time to quit a program. So, let's begin with the first step and take a look at the different levels of sports.

Three Basic Levels of Sports for the Young Athlete

1. Recreational Sports

Recreational sports are run mostly through a city or local group such as a Boys and Girls Club or a YMCA. These sports usually have just one or two practices a week with games on the weekends, and most seasons last six to eight weeks. Often, the coaches are parent volunteers and the atmosphere is less competitive than a "travel team." Of course, you still read about the horror stories of parents losing their mind, assaulting other parents, acting aggressively toward a referee, or screaming at and humiliating their own kid. These incidents involve a miniscule number of people involved in youth sports. It's a real and serious problem, but somehow the headline, "Parents very well-behaved at last week's soccer tournament" doesn't sell as many newspapers.

A recreational league is the best place to start. It's relatively inexpensive and the seasons are long enough to get a taste of the sport, but short enough that if it's not working out it doesn't seem interminable. With such a short season, you aren't likely to see a dramatic improvement in skill, but it will at least allow your kid to see if they like the sport. You'll have the opportunity to notice if they really enjoy it, are sad to see the season end, and show some level of potential.

2. **Competitive Sports**

   Competitive sports often require tryouts, have professional coaches and/or trainers, require a greater number of practices per week, and involve a great deal more expenses (dues, tournament fees, travel expenses, etc.). The first hurdle to participation is making the team. However, if your child has spent time in recreational leagues, you probably have some idea about their ability level. Within the realm of competitive sports, there are different levels and/or clubs whose standards, requirements, and expectations vary. Coaching in competitive sports is often more professional than recreational. Many youth sports teams have excellent, experienced coaches who have been to the highest levels of a sport and know what it takes to get there. Unlike recreational sports, competitive sports have extended seasons, often year-round or close to it. The season is long enough to see substantial improvement, and one year in a competitive atmosphere will often be enough to determine if this is a sport your child wants to pursue.

3. **School Sports**

   School sports generally start as young as fourth grade. Often, the seasons are short and your child could play three or four different sports during a single school year. These teams don't require nearly the same talent and commitment as high school programs and, like recreational programs, offer a chance to gain exposure to a variety of different types of sports. School sports have the added benefit of the camaraderie with other students from the same school.

Four Factors to Consider when Choosing a Program

Once you decide which level of sports is appropriate for your child, it's time to look at specific programs. Even after you join a program, be sure you're constantly evaluating the program to make sure that it still reflects your values. Sports require a significant commitment of time, money, and energy. Be sure that you are making a wise investment.

1. **The Coach**

    In order for your child to have a successful experience in sports, it's extremely important that they have the right coach. As an adult, your job satisfaction can have a great deal to do with your compatibility with your boss. Your child's view of school as a positive or negative experience is greatly influenced by how they relate to their teacher. Similarly, if your child doesn't get along with the coach at all, the chances of long-term success in that sport aren't very good.

    Having a great swim coach as my first experience in sports led me down the path toward being a competitive swimmer. When I look back at all the sports I played, many of them were just "things to do" while they were in season. It was just another basketball season or baseball season. Swimming was different because the coach made it so much fun. It was much more than "just another season"; it captivated me in a way that none of the other sports or coaches were able to, and it became a life-changing experience.

    The role of the coach is so critical to the success of a child athlete that we'll spend an entire chapter discussing it. For now, just keep in mind that it's one of the four important factors to consider when evaluating a program.

2. **Atmosphere**

   Far more important than the actual building or field is the overall atmosphere of the program. Though having good, clean, safe equipment is a major bonus, pay more attention to the general "feel" of the place. Is it a serious program with strict rules, or is the atmosphere relaxed with a focus on having fun? Is it a competitive and goal-oriented atmosphere, or one that's more recreational? If the "win at all costs" mentality hangs over the program and that isn't what you're looking for, then keep looking. Make sure the "feeling" of the program matches up with your goals for your child.

3. **Skill Development**

   Young athletes improve their skills and performance by learning proper technique. Practicing poor shooting form hundreds of times isn't going to make your child a better basketball player. Taking hundreds of wild, uncontrolled swings with a bat isn't going to make your child a better hitter. Swimming up and down the pool doing endless laps with poor form isn't going to make your child a better swimmer. Unfortunately, some programs take the "more is better" approach. This may work for an elite athlete who has spent years perfecting their form and just needs the hundreds and thousands of repetitions required to ingrain the skill into muscle memory. At every age, technique is going to lead to the biggest initial improvement, and then the intensity of the program can be elevated to continue to challenge the athlete. If you want your child to learn or improve a skill, be sure to choose a program that gives attention to technique and form.

4. **Philosophy / Vision**

   You already know what you want your child to get out of the experience. Make sure your expectations match up with that of the coach and program director. Ask the program director what their philosophy is. Ask the coach what they ideally hope the athletes will get out of completing the season. What is the vision for the program, the overall direction that the program hopes to take in the future? How do they see themselves related to the other teams in the area? What makes this team different? Be sure to choose a program whose vision and philosophy are aligned with your own.

When evaluating a program, continually ask yourself the following questions:

- Is the coach a good, positive role model for my child?

- Is this the atmosphere where I want my child to be spending considerable time?

- What is the emphasis of the program? Are they learning / mastering new skills?

- Is the philosophy of the program well stated? Do I agree with it?

- Is there a comprehensive vision for the program? If so, how does my child fit into it?

As Your Child Grows and Changes, the Program Changes

Growing up, I played as many sports as I could. The seasons were fairly short—swimming was in the summer; soccer was ten weeks in the fall and ten weeks in the spring; baseball was ten weeks in the spring; basketball was eight weeks in the winter. It was no problem if the seasons overlapped; in fact, if I didn't have two or three sports going on at the same time, I usually ended up with too much time and energy on my hands. However, each time someone advances in level, the demands of a sport increase and choices have to be made. Swimming went from two times a week to three times a week. I made a travel soccer team and now we had practice twice a week and games on Saturdays. While I found it easy to balance the two sports, it left a little less time for other sports like basketball and baseball.

We moved from Washington, D.C. to Phoenix, AZ when I was ten and that's when the big changes occurred. Swimming went from three times a week for an hour to five times a week for two hours. I could still make soccer work and was able to balance the two, but it became more difficult.

Begin with the end in mind so you can continually make the right decisions as you guide your young athlete.

The payoff was that when I spent more time swimming each week, I got a lot better right away. After just three months, I won the Arizona State Championship for 10 & Unders in two events. This was fun for me because I'd never won anything like that. I also got extremely lucky because I turned eleven the day after the meet. Had my birthday been a couple days earlier, I would have just been in the middle of the pack for eleven- to twelve-year-olds instead of a 10 & Under champion.

Soon after that meet, my swimming career started to falter. All the kids I competed against started growing and I didn't! For the next two years, I barely improved my times. By increasing my practice time three-fold when I was ten, I got the immediate improvement that allowed me to excel against kids who were practicing less, but when the competition began training longer, my advantage was washed away and I never won another state championship.

Rather than quitting, I redoubled my effort and tried to focus on getting better. Fortunately, I was still in soccer and doing very well, so my image of myself as an athlete suffered, but didn't evaporate when I hit the plateau in swimming. Around this time, I also started to get more serious about triathlons, even placing fifth at the National Championship when I was twelve.

When I was thirteen and fourteen, I made minimal improvement in swimming, even though I was doing it every day. I stuck with it because I still had a belief that a major breakthrough was just around the corner. I'd invested so much that I thought I would lose it all if I took a couple months off, or that it would all have been a waste of time if I quit. So, I kept pressing on.

As I turned fifteen, I started to see some measurable improvement, enough for me to go with swimming exclusively when the demands of doing two sports finally caught up to me. After quitting soccer, swimming became a massive

> *The bottom line is this: If your child loves a variety of sports, resist the urge to specialize early.*

commitment. We had practice from 5:10-7:15 four mornings a week, 3:15-6:15 five evenings a week, and Saturday morning from 6-10. Again, once I increased training, my times dropped dramatically. I trained on the above schedule for my last three years of high school. I continued getting more serious about triathlons, spending much of the summer cycling and running and going to races.

There is an inevitable point in the lives of most athletes when they realize that they aren't going to make it to the big time. By the time I was a sophomore in high school, I came to the realization that the only way I was going to make it to the Olympics was to buy a ticket. By the time I was a junior in high school, I realized that I wasn't going to get a college scholarship. At that point, I had to determine what I hoped to get out of swimming and if it was worth it to continue.

I reflected on what had kept me going over the years. First, I always liked my coaches; they made what is otherwise a boring, monotonous activity somewhat fun! Second, I was excited about making it to the next level, especially swimming on the high school and college teams. Third, I liked what it was doing for my body. I had incredible endurance. In soccer, I was the one who never had to come out. My senior year of high school, I ran competitively for the first time and was immediately successful. Most importantly, I had developed an enormous aerobic base without any major injuries. Having this base launched my triathlon career.

Swimming as much as I did set me up for success in high school swimming, college swimming, and triathlon, but I know of many people I swam with who don't hold the same opinion of all the time they spent in the water. It seems that it was only at the end of their swimming career that they took a good look at why they were swimming and what they hoped to get out of it. Many didn't have a good answer. It was just something that they had always done. Many wished that they had tried other things growing up or wished they hadn't gotten quite so serious at such a young age. Others I swam with made the Olympic team and now swim professionally. Swimming is far from a unique example; all sports require a smaller commitment in the beginning, then demand increasingly more with every advancement in level. Begin with the end in mind so you can continually make the right decisions as you guide your young athlete.

Looking back, I didn't really have "the end in mind" at all times. I got discouraged in swimming because I couldn't see the improvement and wasn't sure of the purpose anymore. Because of my personality, I channeled the disappointment into motivation and stuck with it, and became a better person because of it. However, if I had understood the stages of athletic development, I would have had a clearer picture of what I was pursuing.

I was vastly more successful at triathlon than any of the other sports I participated in. It was also the only one I began with the end in mind. My goals in triathlon meant more to me than my goals in the other sports and activities. Gradually, triathlon became the most important activity to me and I made decisions along the way because of that.

The following stages represent a general guideline to help you make decisions as your child grows and changes. Kids don't always operate on a timeline and may move through the stages at different ages. The timeline that follows isn't about goals in any one particular sport. Rather, it's a guide to help you understand the role that sports should be playing at different stages in your child's development. The bottom line is this: If your child loves a variety of sports, resist the urge to specialize early. If they have one sport that stands out above the rest, focus mostly on that sport, but be aware that playing different sports is beneficial because of cross-training and the reduction of the risk of overuse injuries.

Just make sure you resist the idea that your child will be hopelessly behind if they aren't in a league at the youngest age allowed.

The only thing worse than a kid who's totally turned off to sports because they're tired of it by the time they're twelve is the child who's already injured themselves (swimmers shoulder, tennis elbow, baseball elbow, etc.) and is on the road to ruining their body at a young age. Keep in mind that most people have their kids in sports to promote a healthy lifestyle. Too much too soon can be detrimental.

The Five Stages of a Young Athlete

Stage 1: Moving and Learning (Age 5 & Under)

At this age, your primary concern should be finding an activity where your kid is having fun running around. Organized sports aren't critical at this stage because an active four- or five-year-old is probably moving around enough as it is. Organized sports for kids start as young as three years old. Our culture seems to be pushing for more achievement earlier and earlier. What your child did at the age of three on a soccer field or T-ball diamond will not have an effect on the rest of their life. Relax and let them be a child in peace. If they like playing with balls, go into the backyard with them and kick the ball around. Spend some time with your kid and let them just have fun. Very young kids usually lack the coordination to experience any sort of success at activities such as basketball or T-ball, and starting too soon could just lead to frustration.

Do not allow them to give up on sports altogether.

The Exception:

Some children seem to be way too sedentary at a young age, so parents put them in an organized program to get them moving. If your four-or five-year-old is in a program, be sure to explain to them why they're doing it. Many leagues at this age don't keep score and hopefully focus more on playing and learning. Stress over and over that the results don't matter at this age. Lay the foundation for what you expect from them. You can talk about what it means to try your best and be a team player. You can also talk about the rules of a sport, such as what base to run to after you hit the ball. Just make sure you resist the idea that your child will be hopelessly behind if they aren't in a league at the youngest age allowed.

Stage 2: The Big World (Age 6-9)

During this stage, your child will likely play a few different sports. This is not the time to start specializing! It's too early to know what your child is really good at. The two major characteristics that make for a good athlete at this age are size and coordination. If your child is bigger and more coordinated than others their age, they'll likely be good at everything. Sports will come easily to them because they have a huge advantage over the competition. This edge does not last. When other kids start growing and developing greater coordination, the advantage will evaporate.

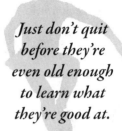

Just don't quit before they're even old enough to learn what they're good at.

If your child is small for their age or uncoordinated, they may not find themselves to be good at anything. If this happens, take a step back. Realize that there still is potential in your child; do not allow them to give up on sports altogether. Try a less competitive program where they'll still get the benefit of fitness while improving their skills, if the competitiveness seems to be a problem. Just don't quit before they're even old enough to learn what they're good at. When they catch up to the other kids in size and coordination, they'll have a great foundation.

Kids should be in many different activities at this stage. They should try everything. They'll start to learn where their strengths are and what activities they most want to pursue. Make fitness a priority, but lay the foundation of skills and techniques in a variety of activities. Their extracurricular activities shouldn't be limited to sports; this is also a great time to learn an instrument or pursue artistic ambitions.

The Exception:

There are certain sports, like gymnastics, which require early specialization. If your child is specializing at this point, be sure to help them keep perspective and stay balanced. If they reach their peak in the given sport in a few years, you don't want them to have to start all over with no experience in anything other than their specialty.

Stage 3: Decision Time (Age 10-12)

This is the stage where, to really excel in a sport, the interest has to be coming from your kid, not solely from you. At this point, it may be apparent that a certain sport just isn't their thing. If the decision is to quit, think through the following question: "Quit to do what?" Make sure there's another activity waiting to take the place. This is an age where physical activity is extremely important; make certain that they do not stop exercising completely. You can decide if sports will become a focus of their childhood or simply remain on the periphery to balance a healthy lifestyle.

> *If the decision is to quit, think through the following question: "Quit to do what?"*

This is also when the demands of everything start coming to a head. More is expected of kids at school and time constraints may force them to give up some activities. After several years of playing lots of different sports, they're starting to get an idea of the sports they like the best and where they have the most potential. At this age, you may start to see them fall behind other kids who are specializing. You may start getting worried that "if they don't make the travel team now, they won't ever be able to break into it." More often than not, it is still too early to specialize in one sport. Before puberty, you cannot know the sport they'll be the best at.

The problem with participating in a sport that requires five practices a week and often has games on the weekends is that the child will not have time (or energy) to pursue any other interests. This may work if the sport has a short season, but sports that require a five-day a week commitment are often year-round sports.

If by the age of ten, your child has already tried every other sport and only likes one, do you pursue that one exclusively? Maybe, but I'd be really careful about that.

> *If they are doing too many activities at this point, they start running the risk of falling behind the kids who are specializing.*

If they're truly enjoying the sport and it's fun for them, you may consider it. But, remember this: You will not be able to get the time back!

My sister Amy was a champion in the breaststroke, but once she hit the age of twelve, she never got another best time in the event. Fortunately for her, she greatly improved her backstroke, ending up with a School Record in high school and a four-year scholarship to the University of Richmond based on her backstroke talent. Swimming is a sport where you have four primary options (strokes) for competition. If her sport had been running and she never got faster after the age of twelve, it would have been a colossal mistake for her to have specialized early and have no other options. The biggest problem with early specialization is that if your child "burns out" (we'll talk about this term later) of a sport at the age of twelve, thirteen, or fourteen, it's going to be very difficult for them to move on to another activity and experience the same level of success they had with their first sport.

Stage 4: Impending Specialization (Age 12-13)

At this point, your child should have a sense of what they're good at, what they enjoy, and what they want to pursue. It's time to consider what the next step is. Do they want to make their high school team, and then their college team? If so, they'll need to do things differently than if they have no such plans.

If they are doing too many activities at this point, they start running the risk of falling behind the kids who are specializing. If they have future aspirations in one sport, doing too many others will risk making them average at all of them and "really good" at none of them. At any age, they will begin to fall behind kids who make one sport their life from the age of seven. However, at this age, they start running out of time to catch up.

There was a swimmer who joined our team in the eighth grade because he wanted to make his high school swim team, which was a very competitive team. Growing up, he had played many sports and was involved in many different activities. Because of the focus of the program he had been swimming with before, his technique was very good. And because he had been exposed to many different sports, he had the necessary strength and endurance. He decided to start swimming at a higher level and within six months he was as fast as I was. At the time, it really bothered me. "How can he be as fast as I am when I've been swimming for so much longer and have worked so much harder?" All through high school, we were about the same speed. His swimming career never launched him to greatness, but because of the background he had in other sports, he was able to get out of swimming what he wanted. I don't think he would have been much faster if he had been swimming seriously since the age of eight; the delayed start didn't hurt him. Because he wasn't already jaded with the sport, he brought eagerness to training that was lacking in the rest of us and was excited by his rapid improvement.

> *If you hope to be an athlete recruited by a college, you must be among the very best in your sport and make a 100 percent commitment to keep yourself there.*

Stage 5: Specialization (Age 14 & Up)
With the end in mind, this is the age to specialize. Some kids who are naturally good at everything may not have to. Jackie Robinson lettered in four sports at UCLA. However, it's exceptionally rare to see even a two-sport athlete at a major college. Because

the sports have become so demanding and specialized, each sport is a fifty-week-a-year commitment. Because so many people specialize, it's harder to jump right in to any sport. If you go to a large high school, it isn't realistic to just play baseball in the spring and expect to make the varsity team. If you hope to be an athlete recruited by a college, you must be among the very best in your sport and make a 100 percent commitment to keep yourself

Refuse to allow them to get down on themselves or start blaming other people (coach, teammates, and referees).

there. If you expect to get a swimming scholarship, you may have to be putting in the thirty hours a week of training in high school that everyone else is doing. When they're awarding college athletic scholarships, they don't give them to the most "well-rounded person." If the goal of your child's athletic participation is an athletic scholarship for college, then they'll have to become extremely good at one sport. As long as they meet the requirements for the university they hope to attend, skill will be primarily what the coach is looking for. However, if that isn't the goal, then make sure your child is enjoying their sport. Sports can certainly be a much more productive use of time than other temptations in high school. At this age, it's still vital to stay active in an enjoyable sport.

So, there you have it, five stages to progress through. To see progress, you have to keep moving! As your child grows up and moves through these stages, they face the inevitable choice of when to get more serious about a sport and when to quit.

When to Jump to the Next Level

Every sport has levels. For some sports, levels are determined strictly by age; for others, ability factors into the equation. How do you know when your child should take it to that next level? At what point should they make the jump from the recreational league to the traveling team? At what point should they advance to the next training group?

First, make sure your child is healthy and physically ready for the next level. Check with a doctor. Also, make sure that your family doctor has some idea of the value that you put on sports. Some of the doctors we had growing up would say things like: "Your shoulders hurt, just stop swimming for three weeks and they'll get better." Others were more realistic and said, "Well, the injury you have isn't very serious, but here are some stretches and exercises you can do to improve strength. Take it easy for the next several days, but you can still keep doing it." If you pile on too much intensity before their body is physically mature enough for it, you're courting disaster.

Mental readiness is as important as physical readiness. If you determine that your child is physically ready, then determine their mental readiness. What you're looking for will depend on their personality. You may have a child who's averse to change and doesn't want to try a "new" group or sport no matter what it is. It might not be time yet to push them forward; you may want to focus on their self-confidence for the time being instead. You may have a child who isn't eager to go to practice anymore; they're not as challenged by it as they used to be because they're getting so much better than the players around them. If it looks like they're not being challenged to develop their skills, they could be ready to make the jump.

Often, the time will just "feel right" to go for it. Your child might be excited about the prospect of advancing or they many not be. Again, know your child well enough to be able to read if this is something that they would be excited about once they were doing it. Every time they advance a level, you must be prepared for an increase in time, energy, and money spent on the activity. Often it's very worthwhile, but if they aren't excited about it, don't have goals in the sport, and don't seem to be "getting more into it," then the time might not be right.

If you decide your child should advance, be ready to help them make the adjustment. It

> *"Most people fail instead of succeed because they trade what they want most for what they want at the moment."*

could mean going from being the star of the recreational league to spending a lot of time on the bench in the competitive league. It could mean going from being the best in their training group to being forced to work tirelessly while falling behind. This is a great opportunity to reinforce what it means to be part of the team. Talk with them about having to "earn" playing time and a starting position. What are their ideas about what it will take to get back into the starting line-up or back at

Pay more attention to your child's demeanor after a practice than before it.

their favorite position? Refuse to allow them to get down on themselves or start blaming other people (coach, teammates, and referees).

When to Quit

Every athlete has days when they want to quit. Everyone has days when they don't want to go to practice or don't want to go to a game. But as Lance Armstrong said: "If you never quit when the going got tough, you wouldn't have anything to regret for the rest of your life."

On the ceiling above my bed hangs a quote: "Most people fail instead of succeed because they trade what they want most for what they want at the moment." How true is this statement? Its veracity extends far beyond sports. If you have a goal and a plan to reach that goal, you know what you should be doing "at the moment" whatever that moment might be. The reason I keep that quote above my bed is so that it's the first thing I see when I wake up every morning. In the summers, I'm usually up by 4:00 a.m. and out the door training by 4:30, six days a week. It's the only way to get training done in Phoenix where we routinely can hit a hundred degrees by 8:00 a.m. When my alarm rudely interrupts my sleep at the obscene hour of 4:00 a.m., what do I want most? It's always the same answer: to finish on the podium at the Hawaii Ironman Triathlon. What do I want at the moment? To turn off the alarm and go back to sleep. The days where I bound out of bed eager to jump on my bike for a five-hour ride aren't as common as one would hope. I usually have to drag myself out of bed; yet five minutes into the ride, I love it.

That's my mental battle every morning and I'm doing this for a living. I'd be amazed at the kid who never complains about going to practice. Think about your own life. Don't you have days where you don't want to go to the gym or just feel like skipping work? It doesn't mean that you don't ever want to work out or that you want to quit your job—it just means that you're having "one of those days."

Pay more attention to your child's demeanor *after* a practice than *before* it. I hear the following observation from parents all the time: "She complains about going to practice all the way there, but once she's there she loves it." Sounds just like my getting out of bed and on the bike.

On the other hand, a major red flag would be if they were excited to go to practice, then depressed after practice. It's fine for them to be tired, it's OK to have worked harder than they thought possible and explored the limits of their potential. However, if the "downer" after practice is more than just harmless fatigue, and the joy that's there when going to practice is sucked out by the end of the session, there may be something wrong. Also, see if the same disposition is related to other activities. Do they have a hard time going to school, to band, to scouts or other activities they previously enjoyed? If they're losing interest in everything, it may be a sign that they're overscheduled and need to drop something.

If the problem is specific to a certain sport and the complaining is consistent before and after practice, try to narrow down the problem. Is it a problem with the coach? Is it a problem with other players on the team? Are they just sick of the sport? The single most important question to ask when they want to quit is: "Quit to do what?" If the answer is quit to do another sport or because they are

> *The single most important question to ask when they want to quit is: "Quit to do what?" If the answer is quit to do another sport or because they are hopelessly behind at school, that's one thing. If it's quit so they can sit home, watch television, and play video games, that's quite another.*

hopelessly behind at school, that's one thing. If it's quit so they can sit home, watch television, and play video games, that's quite another.

Children shouldn't be forced to do a particular sport, but they should be forced to do something. Sitting at home all the time cannot be an option. Would their attitude be any different if they were doing a different sport that required a similar level of exertion? Do they not like the coach, the team, or the sport? If they don't like the sport and refuse to put in a minimum level of effort, would a different sport produce different results?

Unless they're in a dangerous or destructive atmosphere, do not let them quit in the middle of a season. Talk to them about the commitment they made to the team and to themselves when they signed up. Besides, you need to give it a full season before they have the full experience of the sport. After the season, then it's time to evaluate whether they want to continue or try something else.

Chapter Summary

Once you look at your child's personality and decide what you hope for them to get out of sports, the next step is to find the right activity and program. This is an ongoing process and you should be prepared for some trial and error. You're looking to find an eventual "good fit" between your child and the activity they choose or you choose for them.

1. Choose the right level based on what your child needs.
   - Recreational
   - Competitive
   - School Sports

2. Choose the right program, considering the following factors:
   - Coach
   - Atmosphere
   - Skill Development
   - Philosophy/Vision

3. Understand that the right fit for your child depends on their physical, mental, and emotional maturity level.

4. If the answer is ever to quit, be sure to have an answer for this question: "Quit to do what?"

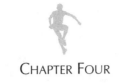

CHAPTER FOUR

CHAPTER FOUR

COACH AND TEAM DYNAMICS

Joe's Rule #4: "The coach matters more than the sport."

Having your child coached by the right person and on the right team is much more important than what sport they are playing. As kids age and begin to push their boundaries, they usually want to listen to their parents less and less. When they don't want to listen to their parents anymore, they'll often listen to their friends—which can be good or bad, depending on the friends. They also listen to their coaches. Is your child's coach someone you believe will counter the daily wave of negativity? Do you trust your child's coach to be a positive role model? If you don't have a crystal clear understanding of what your child hopes to get out of sports and what you expect from the coach and team you choose, you and your child may not be happy with the experience.

The "right fit" for your child, the coach they play for and the team they play with, will depend on what you want out of the experience. Again, there aren't too many bad coaches or bad teams out there. But not every coach and team is right for every child.

Guidelines for Choosing a Coach and Team

In Chapter 2, we looked at a number of reasons children play sports. Those reasons fall into the following three categories. Your child's reason for participation will determine which route to go when choosing a coach and team. The reasons may overlap but are not mutually exclusive.

If your goal is: Participation for Health

Even if your child isn't an athlete, they need to play sports. Health, as used in this context, is the absence of disease. Participation for health means that you're doing just enough to avoid the health risks that come from inactivity. You don't really care too much how they perform or if they improve their skills in a particular sport, you just want to keep them away from the television.

Go this route if:

You just need to get your child off the couch and into something athletic. Do this if they are averse to competition. Don't be afraid to try several different sports. The more you try, the more chance you have of finding one they like. Once you've found a sport that's a good fit, think about finding a league or team that will allow your child to thrive.

What to look for in a coach and team:

Choose a non-competitive program. Choose a sport where your child can get a lot of activity. The coach you're looking for is one who can make the sport fun. An extensive background in the sport isn't necessary; you're looking for someone who makes the task of coming to practice and being active a little less traumatic for the otherwise couch potato.

If your goal is: Participation for Fitness

Participation for fitness means that you want your child doing more than the minimum. There is a competitive element beginning to come into play because when you do a sport for fitness reasons, you start to want to do it better than the people around you, or at least better than your previous performances. You're not only interested in your child being healthy (absence of disease), but also looking for improvement in performance. You want them to master the skills present in the sport.

Go this route if:

You aren't sure where to start or you want to see how your child responds to a sport before going further into a competitive league. This is also a good choice if they love a sport, but don't want it to consume all of their free time.

What to look for in a coach and team:

Choose a coach and team whose focus is on technique and skill development. The way for a young athlete to maximize their potential is by mastering the fundamentals. As they gain size and strength, their performance will improve (though not always at a linear rate) as long as the foundation is solid.

If your goal is: Participation for Performance

Participation for performance means that you want your child doing everything possible to be the best they can be at a given activity. This is almost exclusively the realm of competitive sports. Participation for performance means going for the win. It means cuts for the kids who aren't good enough "right now" for this level of competition. It means playing the best players at the games, which means time on the bench for the less talented athletes. If you push your child onto a competitive team before their skills are at that level, they will continually measure up short against their more talented peers. At a younger age, it's much better for them to be on a less competitive team where they have a chance to play and be successful than on a more competitive team where they'll be sitting on the bench.

Go this route if:

Your child has tried lower levels of a sport and needs the next step. Make sure it's a sport they truly love and you're convinced that it isn't just a passing interest. This level of commitment will require making sacrifices in other activities.

What to look for in a coach and team:

Look for a dedicated team and a coach who will be able to get through to your child. Make sure the coach is someone who's balanced and keeps perspective because this is the model where a dramatic increase of youth sports injuries is beginning to be seen. Though training for performance can be positive, you must make absolutely certain that you have the right coach. The risks are too great and the stakes are too high.

Make sure that you aren't part of the problem. I've talked to a number of physical therapists who see kids with injuries, and their parents are expecting a miracle so that "Johnny will be able to pitch on Sunday." There is no game that's important enough to justify risking permanent damage to a growing body.

Technique at this level is of utmost importance; coaches must be skilled. Participation for performance requires a great deal of repetition. If young athletes are repeating a skill (throwing a baseball, running, hitting a tennis ball) over and over with poor technique, the risk of injury greatly escalates. Poor coaching can result in overuse injuries. A good athlete, a good coach, and a good parent understand that no medal, trophy, or youth sports championship is worth risking a debilitating injury.

If you don't match your child's level of commitment with the right team, they won't have a positive experience. You want your child to be surrounded by a like-minded team. If all you and your child really care about is participation for health and your child ends up on a team where the coach is training the kids for performance, the situation will be frustrating for everyone. If your child is motivated by competition and has a tremendous drive to improve and be the best at a sport, they won't be happy if they're surrounded by kids who are just there for the exercise.

Once you determine your goals for participation, you need to find the coach and the team that will complement this. It's an ongoing process.

What to Look for in a Coach

1. **Is the coach a Parent Volunteer Coach or a Paid Coach?**

    If you're just signing your kid up to play soccer in the city league, you usually won't have a choice of coaches. However, you can start paying attention to the way coaches interact with their players and see what works best with your child. Volunteer coaches are mostly in recreational leagues. A volunteer coach is coaching for one of several reasons. Often they have a child on the team. Or, they may really have a love for the game and a desire to teach it to the next generation. Once the season begins, there is no opportunity to change coaches or teams, so whatever the situation is, you need to make the best of it. Your child may have a different coach every season; it's a good opportunity for them to experience different types of instruction and learn to respond to different authority figures.

    A professional coach is paid, and with the compensation comes added expectations. Coaching is an interesting profession. Anyone can call themselves a coach; often, you don't need any sort of certification to begin coaching. Sports that do require certification generally look at safety credentials (CPR, First Aid, etc.) rather than any sort of competency in the sport for initial certification. Competitive teams or "club" teams or "travel" teams will often have professional coaches. These people usually have extensive experience in the sport, but not necessarily. One of my favorite swim coaches in high school had a rowing background and never swam competitively himself. He's coached numerous Olympians and held high profile leadership positions in three different countries. A professional coach is often the one coaching a team that requires a great time commitment. It is extremely important that they understand the physiology of young athletes and that they're able to instruct them to perform the skills properly so as to lessen the risk of injury.

2. **How well does the coach teach the sport?**

It doesn't take much to say things like "run faster" and "keep your eye on the ball." How does the coach *teach* these skills? Can the coach relate well enough to the children so that they understand what the coach is saying and are able to improve their skills? A good coach and a good teacher have a lot in common.

In the seventeen years I was a competitive swimmer, I swam at a number of different levels and had about two dozen different coaches. Some of them were Olympic gold medalists; others had no competitive swimming experience of their own. Being a good athlete and being a good coach require two different sets of skills. Some of the best coaches I had struggled in their own swimming career because it didn't come easily to them. They had to work for everything they attained and knew what it felt like to "not get it." It reminded me of a friend of mine who was struggling in his Calculus class in college. My friend said that the professor was such a genius, even multivariable calculus came easily to him—he just couldn't understand how anyone could struggle with basic calculus. Sometimes the best teachers are those who had the same struggles with the material they have to help their students master. If a person is coaching a sport that came easily to them, it may be more difficult to teach it.

> *What matters more in a coach at the youth level is how well they can teach your child, not necessarily what they themselves accomplished as an athlete.*

Therein lies the big divide between being a great player and a great coach. The great player needs to be able to "do" and "show." The star player has to perform under pressure and come through for the team when that all-star performance is needed. They also need to be able to "show" so they can help the team. They can give pointers to other players on the team who are close to their level and understand the intricacies of the sport. A great coach, especially at the youth level, needs to be able to teach and lead. The "teaching" part is very different from "showing." With "showing," you're demonstrating to someone with major skill already present how to take it up a notch. With "teaching," you're taking someone who's very new to the sport or activity and getting them started with a basic set of skills.

While it's important that the coach's style works for your child, remember that learning how to get along with coaches and teachers is a great life skill.

Now, a great player and a great coach are certainly not mutually exclusive. There are many great players who went on to be great coaches. If you can find a great coach who was also a great player, there's the added benefit of the coach knowing what it takes to reach that highest level and providing a constant reminder to your child that greatness in the sport is possible. In fact, it's right in front of them. What matters more in a coach at the youth level is how well they can teach your child, not necessarily what they themselves accomplished as an athlete.

3. **Does the coach's style work for your child?**

   Every coach has a different style. I always have fun while I'm coaching. That's part of my style. I got tired of hearing my kids complain that the water was cold when it was eighty-four degrees, so I told them that when I was their age we had to break the ice off the pool with a hammer before we got in. By the time they finished telling me what a liar I was and carrying on about how that wasn't possible, they had forgotten about the allegedly "cold" water. I countered by saying they weren't even alive back when I was their age, so they would have no idea what the world was like—it was a very different place. I had successfully taken their focus off of themselves and put it on me.

Try to find a coach who will connect with your child.

This distraction technique worked and I soon extended it to cover any possible complaint they could come up with. If they complained about their toe hurting, I told them of the time I had my leg chopped off at the knee and had to tape it back on with duct tape before practice. When they complain about school, I tell them about the time I had to do a book report on the dictionary in second grade: "It took forever to read—it had, like, no plot and jumped around a lot." This was back when we would have to walk four miles through the snow barefoot—to and from school, uphill both ways. They do a lot less complaining now because I always launch into my long-winded recounting of how things were so much more difficult and "kids these days don't appreciate anything." By the time they stop laughing at me and telling me they don't care what things were like back then and I'm the "biggest liar in the world," they move beyond their momentary complaint and get back into the groove of a good practice.

As I said, each coach has their own style. Notice the coach's style and whether or not it works for your child. If your child complains about the coach's style, before letting them focus on the negative, encourage your child to see if there's anything they can learn from the coach. Chances are you won't always like the way your boss leads. If you want to stay at the job, you'd better change your outlook. While it's important that the coach's style works for your child, remember that learning how to get along with coaches and teachers is a great life skill.

4. **Does your child connect with the coach?**

I learned early on in my college years that the professor was a lot more important than the course. A great professor could take the most boring of subjects and bring it to life. The reverse, unfortunately, is also true. A professor has the ability to suck the life out of an otherwise interesting subject. I filled my entire religion minor taking classes from one professor. There was something about Ron Miller's teaching style that really captivated me. We weren't assigned a textbook and asked to recite information he had presented or we had read. Instead, all of our reading was from primary sources, the actual work of theologians, and we were required to analyze and synthesize the information. We were to go beyond the scope of the book to apply the truths within to other situations. Perhaps you had a teacher like that? One whose name, face, and voice you still can recall. Something they said or did connected with you on a basic level. I chose my elective classes based more on the professor than the course description. An inept professor could make the most interesting material intolerable just as an outstanding professor could bring the dullest of material to life. A great coach works the same way.

You can't overestimate the importance of a good coach at a young age. My first coach was Phil Levine. When I was five, I believed that I could do anything that my sister Amy could do. She signed up for a diving class at the local pool, so I did the same. I had no fear of jumping off the one-meter diving board and thought maybe I could learn how to dive off it. It was then that I met Phil Levine; he became my diving coach and was probably the person outside of my immediate family who had the most impact on my early life. I have recently talked to Phil about the events I describe and he doesn't remember them nearly as vividly as I do. For him, it was just another day on the job; for me, it was a day I'll never forget.

On the last day of the diving class, Phil said that I needed to walk to the top of the three-meter board with him. Now this board was about ten feet high, much higher than the board I was used to. He promised me that I didn't have to go off the board, I just had to walk up to the top and see how high it was. As I stood at the end of the board looking down at how far the water below was, he had me put my hands over my head, then pushed me off. I did an amazing belly flop. Another kid may have reacted differently to being pushed off the board, but my coach knew me and knew what he was doing. I still remember how much it hurt, but after a couple minutes, the pain wore off and I realized it wasn't so bad. I tried it again. Then again. I dove off the three-meter board about a dozen times that day. By the end of the summer, I was running from one end of the board to the other and taking flying leaps off, then executing pretty good dives. Not too bad for a five-year-old. This is one of those early lessons that stuck with me. None of my friends could even dive off the lower board. I realized that just because other people my age couldn't do something or didn't want to do something didn't mean that I couldn't.

The next year, Phil Levine became the coach of the Brookfield Breakers Summer Swim Team and started coaching me in swimming instead of diving. This is where my love for the sport of swimming really developed. Long after that, I realized that my early love for the sport had more to do with the coach than with the sport itself. I believe that had Phil been a bowling coach instead of a swim coach, I would be a pro bowler rather than a professional triathlete.

Try to find a coach who will connect with your child. Different children will respond differently to the same situation. Children have different needs when it comes to coaching, which is why there is no one perfect coach or one particular style to which everyone will respond the best. Your child's personality will determine what type of coach will be the best fit. Just because you disagree with a coach's philosophy doesn't mean that it's wrong—it just means that it's not right for you or your child.

5. **How does the coach motivate the players?**

   Every team has days when things just aren't going right. What does the coach do to get the team back on track? On days when practice is going well, what does the coach do to make the most of the momentum? How does the coach turn a practice into a learning experience? What do they do to make the kids want to improve for their own sake? Look for a coach who knows how to motivate your child.

6. **How does the coach interact with others (players / parents / officials)?**

   Is the coach modeling good behavior? How does the coach react when dealing with the players and their parents? Is their attitude at games appropriate? A good coach doesn't try to please everyone. Robert Frost said, "I don't know the secret of success, but I know the secret to failure is to try to please everyone." You can't expect that everyone will be happy all of the time. Look for a coach who treats players, parents, and officials with respect and expects the same in return.

7. **Why is the coach coaching?**

   It's also important to get a sense of what motivates your child's coach. Coaching isn't a high-paying job. Why do they do it? If you aren't sure, then ask. If they don't know, that's not a good sign. I coach because I see how having an outstanding coach at an early age transformed my life. Coaching isn't about me. I tell people that my massive ego is satisfied by my success in the sport of triathlon. I'm not living through the kids I coach; their performance is about them, it's not about me. I'm not trying to advance myself at the expense of my athletes; I just want them to achieve their personal goals and live a healthy, fulfilling life.

   A lot of coaches (especially ones in individual sports) are looking for that one great athlete who will put them on the map—the "Carmichael phenomenon." Chris Carmichael was the personal coach of Lance

Armstrong. Chris Carmichael is, no doubt, a great cycling coach, but he became famous because of his work with Armstrong. Some coaches are latching onto younger and younger kids and trying to build their name alongside (sometimes at the expense of) the athlete.

Be aware of coaches who focus only on the kids who are winning at a young age. If your child isn't yet a great baseball player, doesn't have the arm or the strength of his teammates, but has excellent fundamentals, he's going to vastly improve. But in the meantime, the coach may overlook him. Once his development catches up to the rest of the kids, he could have laid the foundation of technique and surpass those kids who had early success because of their size, strength, and coordination. By emphasizing results instead of processes and by focusing too much on stats and results too early, certain types of coaches don't give the players who have potential as much opportunity.

What to Look for in a Team

A great team inspires all of its members to new heights. The more commitment a sport requires, the more time your child will spend with the team. I've been on some great teams and some terrible teams. It's said that there is nothing more frustrating than having a great performance on a day when your team loses. I guess that's one of the things that led me into individual sports. I got to the point where it really bothered me that other people on my team didn't care about the game as much as I did. I was tired of having the outcome hanging in the balance while someone who was always messing around at practice consistently came up short when it mattered.

Your child is not a professional – remember that!

When choosing a team or deciding whether your child should continue with a team, there are some specific things you need to look at.

1. **The Team Atmosphere**

   What kind of kids make up the team and how do they interact with each other? Does the coach command and receive respect? Do the kids genuinely seem to support each other and work together toward the good of the team? Every team has rough days, especially as kids hit the middle school years and are engulfed by change. Notice whether the kids spend their time building each other up or tearing each other down.

   No college coach and no professional scout is ever going to care if your child was a state champion when they were ten years old.

2. **Emphasis of the Program**

   What seems to be the most important thing to the team? Are the team's priorities the same as the parents' and the coach's? An optimally functioning team has everyone on board. It's up to the coach to show leadership and present a direction for the program. Is the emphasis on winning, personal improvement, or having fun? Those are all good goals, but everyone has to share the same vision. Does the program seek to instill values that go beyond the boundaries of the playing field? If so, how are those values presented?

3. **Schedule**

   The schedule will give you a very good idea of what's important to the team. Make sure you understand the commitment the team is asking for and be sure your child can live up to those expectations. One parent told me that his ten-year-old daughter's soccer team wanted permission to play in four tournaments on consecutive weekends after the season was over. It would mean approximately sixteen games in twenty-two days. He compared the situation with his oldest daughter who was playing in college on scholarship—her entire season was eighteen games over two and a half months.

There are leagues that demand high levels of commitment, and there are leagues that have one practice and one game a week. There's also a lot in between. Make sure that the schedule of the team fits with your child's goals.

Your Role as a Parent

For a coach to be successful instructing young athletes, they must be able to teach the fundamentals of the sport and somehow make the sport fun. Coaches have their job, and you have yours. Remember that you are the parent and the coach is the coach. There are a handful of high profile "sports parents" who are overly involved in the careers of their children. This phenomenon is mostly seen in individual sports. It's these parents who get significant media coverage, so people tend to forget there are parents of other star athletes who don't share their child's spotlight. For every Earl Woods (father of Tiger Woods) or Richard Williams (father of Venus and Serena Williams), there are countless other parents who backed off and their children became great athletes, like Amy Van Dyken.

The following are tips for how to be a good sports parent:

1. **Don't treat your child like a professional athlete.**

    We all admire athletes like Curt Schilling who pitched in the World Series with a serious ankle injury, or Kerri Strug who completed her final vault with a severely sprained ankle in the 1996 Olympics. But your child is not a professional; remember that! To be a professional athlete means making decisions that sacrifice health in return for optimal performance in a single sport. Do not treat your child like a professional athlete. Much is made of Olympic swimmer Michael Phelps training every day, not even taking Christmas off. While that may be appropriate for a professional athlete, it does not translate to

I didn't have one college coach who, in the recruiting process, said: "Tell me about the races you won when you were ten or twelve."

youth sports. When Michael Phelps was an age-group swimmer, he wasn't swimming every day.

No college coach and no professional scout is ever going to care if your child was a state champion when they were ten years old. I should know. I was one. I won the Arizona State Championship in two swimming events at the 1991 State championship meets. Guess what? Nobody cared. I didn't have one college coach in the recruiting process say: "Tell me about the races you won when you were ten or twelve." No college admissions officer ever said: "Joe, tell me about your report cards when you were in fourth grade." Is it important to do well in school in fourth grade? Sure, because it sets the stage and ingrains the habits that will lead to continued success at the higher levels. You want your fourth grader to do well in school so they

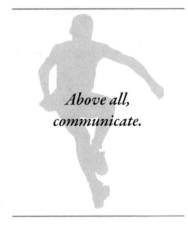

Above all, communicate.

understand the process of learning, build the foundation of future success, and develop a lifelong love of learning, not because something they learn in fourth grade is going to make a difference twenty years from now.

2. **Be patient and positive.**

Help your child look beyond today toward his or her goals. Recognize that athletes develop at different paces, but all athletes need encouragement. No matter how your child seems to be doing in comparison to other athletes, don't heap pressure on them. When they're ready, the big improvement will come. Help your child to be positive and supportive of their teammates; this will lead to a strong sense of sportsmanship and a positive self-image.

3. **Recognize that "The Coach is the Coach."**

   Once you've found a coach you and your child are comfortable with, then back off! You must trust the coach to do what is right for the player and the team. If you can't trust the coach, then find another one. You should consider the field or court a classroom. During a practice, if the coach isn't talking to the athletes, they're analyzing, thinking, and watching. If you have a question, ask it after practice. Treat a coach with the same respect you would give a teacher. You wouldn't go into a classroom and tell the teacher that they're doing their job all wrong.

   Above all, communicate. If you question any aspect of the sports program, make an appointment and discuss it with the coach. If you have a question about what a coach is doing at a practice or a game, go ahead and ask it. Choose a time when they'll be able to give you their attention, not during a practice or a game. Questions like, "What's wrong with you? Why aren't you playing my kid?" are generally unproductive. Something like, "What does Johnny specifically need to work on in order to improve so he can contribute more to the team?" is better.

4. **Prepare your child for success off the field.**

   To increase your child's chances for success on the field, make sure you're meeting their needs off the field. Make sure they're eating right, drinking enough, and getting enough sleep. Make sure their academic obligations are met and that they're still enjoying what they're doing. Simply put, to be a good sports parent, you must be a good parent. Your child needs to know they're safe with you and that no matter their performance on the field, you still love them.

5. **Help your child understand that it won't always be fun.**

   Some days you probably love your job, and some days you may hate your job. You don't just up and quit if things are tough at work for a month. Kids need to understand that. There are going to be times that are very difficult, especially in the beginning of a season. Take a second look if this lack of fun in the sport persists and try to find the root of it. But don't go rushing in to solve problems that may not truly exist. Sometimes time is the best doctor.

Time will tell how much your child's moods affect their interest in a sport. *Temporary motivation* is often the result of a child being *inspired*. Something sparks their interest (their best friend is playing a certain sport and loving it) and they become motivated as a result. But moods can easily affect this kind of motivation, getting in the way and making it short-lived. This is when it's particularly important for a child to understand that "it won't always be fun." When a child is *permanently motivated*, they usually don't see a bad day or a disappointing game as a reason to quit; this type of motivation is more long-term and self-sustaining.

Inspiration is something that happens to someone, and motivation is something that happens *through* someone. Inspiration comes from the outside. You won't ever hear someone say, "I'm such an inspiration to myself." In contrast, motivation can only come from *within*. Motivation is what carries someone through the hardships they confront while pursuing a goal. Motivation is what is left after the inspiration fades.

6. **Help your child understand that it's OK to try things they aren't comfortable with.**

   I spent a great deal of time in this chapter talking about how to find a coach and a team that you're comfortable with. While comfort is very important, don't discourage your child from moving outside their comfort zone for a season. It's OK to give something a try, even if they aren't too sure it's going to work out perfectly. The worst that can happen is that the season will be a loss and they'll move on to another team at the first opportunity. Don't necessarily wait until everything is perfect, because that time may never come.

7. **Help your child understand that it's OK to feel discouraged and defeated.**
    There will be days when something that the coach did or said or something that happened with a teammate frustrates your child. They may be upset with their performance or discouraged because everyone seems better than them. Again, give them some time to bounce back. Many times, great lessons are learned by failing. They will manage their adversity and come back stronger. Kids don't need their parents to bail them out of every little discomfort.

8. **If you aren't sure what to do, just do something.**
    Something is almost always better than nothing. Get your child involved. If all else fails and you can't decide between two alternatives, then flip a coin. If, while the coin is in the air, you find yourself hoping that one side comes up, then you've made your decision.

Chapter Summary

Your child will be the most successful if they're playing a sport they love for a coach they respect on a team they feel a part of. Even if it's not the ideal environment, they'll continue to be active and learn new skills. Continually evaluating your child's coach, team, and program is an ongoing process, one well worth your time.

CHAPTER FIVE

MOTIVATION

▲

Joe's Rule #5: "To reach their full potential, they must want it for themselves."

Motivation is the single most important factor in your child's success or failure in sports. Skills can be taught, but if your child isn't motivated, they won't reach their fullest potential. Motivation isn't a toggle switch. There isn't just "motivated" and "unmotivated," "on" or "off." Like many other attributes, their motivation will rest somewhere on a spectrum between very motivated and completely unmotivated.

Motivation, as I'm referring to it, is the inward desire to succeed at a given task. Motivation isn't something that can be forced on someone; they have to want it for themselves. First you need to have answered the following questions: "To what end?" and "What is the right program for my child?" It's difficult to be motivated if you don't know why you're doing what you're doing and you have no goals. It's also difficult to be motivated if you're in a sport or level of a sport that isn't compatible with your goals.

In order for someone to "be motivated," they have to have a perceived need and become excited to fulfill that need. To understand motivation, you must accurately

> *Success must be defined not as outdoing the efforts of others, but surpassing one's own goals.*

define success. Success must be defined not as outdoing the efforts of others, but surpassing one's own goals. That's what makes setting goals, specifically personal goals, so important. Without a goal in mind, motivation becomes very difficult, if not impossible. Each child will have different goals based on what motivates them, so let's look at some types of motivation.

Types of Motivation

People are motivated by a need to feel successful, to achieve a meaningful end. Each child has a different internal definition of success. One child may define success internally and continually strive to become the best they can be. Another child may define success as getting through the day by expending the least possible effort. Obviously, it's much more difficult to motivate the second child to do something productive. Take a look at the following examples and take note of what motivates your child so you can determine how to help them fulfill that need through their athletic participation.

1. **Friendship**

   For some, the opportunity to hang out with kids their own age is motivation enough to continue participation in sports. Motivation for success at a particular activity could be in the form of recognition and acceptance from their peer group.

2. **Awards**

   Building an ever-increasing trophy/medal/ribbon collection is motivation for some. In sports, medals and trophies are often used as external rewards. While a fine motivator initially, the child who is doing an activity only for the trophy at the end of the year or the medal that will come with a good performance at the end of the season, will soon find that they need more and more to stay satisfied. The "awards junkie" will never truly get their fix. It's important that your child understands that the medal isn't important in itself, but rather the value of the experience represented by the medal that's important.

Talk with your child about what each piece of their collection means to them. What did they learn in the season or competition where they won that medal? Eventually, the motivation must be internalized and the sense of pride that comes from having goals and following through on them will outweigh the value placed on a plastic trophy, a blue ribbon, or a gold-painted medal.

3. **Personal Improvement**

   The knowledge that they're improving their skills and getting better at a particular activity can provide sufficient motivation for some children. If this is your child's motivation, you can help them by keeping their focus on the process of skill development and pointing out when their performance shows improvement.

4. **Praise**

   Encouragement and recognition can be an extremely important source of motivation for some. However, true self-esteem and the kind of confidence that doesn't easily disappear can only be earned, not given. While it's certainly helpful to receive praise, you don't want your child needing it all the time and unable to perform without it.

5. **Competition**

   The thrill of competition, and the need to continue this experience of excitement is something that keeps a certain type coming back for more. These children have a higher internal set-point and have a stronger need for the adrenaline rush and the endorphin high. They're continually on a quest for excitement.

6. **Rewards**

   Some kids are motivated by a reward system set up by their parents. While this can be effective, it's best to reward the process rather than the result, especially if the child doesn't have control over the result.

Rewarding results can have troublesome consequences. Offering them money for each goal they score is not a good idea because it doesn't promote team play. It also has the risk of dependency. This should be something that they do anyway, not because you're paying them for it; dad promising them five dollars shouldn't really be a factor. Paying a bonus for winning a race is similarly a bad idea because the child can't control the rest of the field. Sports at the youth level should be about process and development, not strictly about results. Keep in mind the big picture: When your child finally hangs up the towel for the final time, scores will mean nothing and the whole reason you put your child in the sport will emerge and be a large part of their success and personality.

When you reward the process and not just the result, you're moving from a situation where you're just bribing them to perform to one where they can experience delayed gratification by earning something they desire through hard work and dedication. Sound familiar? It should. You've probably been doing it your whole life.

If you decide to set up a rewards system, it should be reasonable, enforceable, process-oriented, and temporary. Even the best systems can only be effective short term.

In a perfect world, everyone would be motivated intrinsically. That is, they would do the right thing simply because it was the right thing to do. But that's not always how it works. Many smart employers offer bonuses to their employees. For example, if you meet your sales quota for the year, you get a $10,000 bonus. That's external motivation for you. They don't expect you to make your quota just because it's what's best for the company; sometimes external gratification helps motivate you to perform your job to the best of your abilities. There's no right or wrong motivation, but the more you can help your child develop intrinsic motivation, the more you're setting them up for true personal success.

Now that we've taken a look at some different types of motivation, let's look at the various levels of motivation that can be seen in the different motivation personalities.

Types of Motivation Personalities

While one child may be motivated by awards and another may be motivated by competition, there are also differences between how motivated each child is and how short-term or long-term their motivation

Because staying active is vital for every child.

tends to be. Understanding your child's motivation personality will help you guide them through their different stages of athletic participation.

1. **The Flameout**

   This individual is excited about trying something new, but as soon as they run into some difficulty, they're ready to bail. This unhealthy pattern is fed by our "instant gratification" culture. Watching the Olympics on TV or going to a professional sporting event may inspire them. Maybe they have friends who are playing a certain sport. They're really excited to begin, but as soon as they hit a rough spot, they want to quit. Maybe something came very easily to them in the beginning, but as soon as they saw the kind of work that would be required to move from "good" to "great," it scared them off. Maybe they dominated a recreational basketball league, but once they moved up to a more competitive league, they found out that they weren't the star and wanted to quit.

   Dealing with The Flameout Personality

   Life is a difficult game. Help your child build resiliency by allowing them to fail and rebuild. A knockdown isn't a knockout if you get up. Sports provide a great opportunity to learn this vital life lesson. Nothing worthwhile ever comes easily. Any sports star can tell you about times they fell flat on their face. It doesn't mean your child has to stick with every activity they don't like; just don't let quitting in the face of adversity become a habit. Think about times in your own life when you didn't get what you wanted right away. Even if you never reached a particular goal, the amount you likely learned in the process was well worth the sacrifice.

2. The Slow to Warm Up

This type doesn't want to try anything new. If you ask them if they want to do something, the answer is usually "no." However, once you finally drag them to it, they like it and are excited about their new activity.

Dealing with the Slow to Warm Up Personality

With this personality type, you need to continually remind them of their past successes. They tend to be afraid of new experiences, particularly afraid of failure. You need to get them to focus more on enjoyment of the activity. Once they establish a level of comfort, they enjoy it. It's not that they don't want to do anything, they just need a little bit more of a push to get started.

3. The Optimally Motivated

New tasks and challenges excite this individual. They have specific goals in their activities and have a spark of excitement whenever they play. With this one, the biggest challenge is holding them back from overdoing it.

Dealing with the Optimally Motivated Personality

The motivated child is excited by life and really wants to do well. Still the challenge remains in selecting activities that will allow them to maintain or grow their interest, even holding them back if the situation calls for it. This is a very driven child, and you need to encourage balance and healthy participation by helping them set limits when necessary. It's also very important to focus that motivation into goals that will channel their unbridled excitement into success—however they define success. Keep tabs on their feeling toward their sport; notice if there are any changes in motivation. Everything is cyclical. It's nearly impossible to maintain a motivational peak. There will be rises and falls in the motivation level. Don't worry too much about a disposition on a particular day; instead, look for trends that are indicative of larger behavior patterns.

4. **The Under-Motivated**

This type seems to always want the "maximum minimum." They don't appear to be motivated by very much, at least not in the realm of sports.

Dealing with the Under-Motivated Personality

First, determine if this lack of motivation is strictly related to sports. Are they motivated in other areas of life? If your child shows a keen sense of motivation in other areas (school, music, art, etc.) and just hates sports, then you'll have to work a little harder to find a physical activity they do like. Let them try a couple different teams. Give them some choices: "Do you want to do swimming, soccer, or basketball this spring?" "None of the above" is not one of the options. Eventually something will click. They'll find a sport they enjoy, a group of friends they want to continue to be with, or a coach they like to play for.

Even when they find a sport, team, or coach they like, you may notice that the under-motivated child still doesn't want to go to practice sometimes. If you're wondering why, it's probably the same reason that you don't always want to go to the gym after work. They may have had a long day and are tired. Going home and sitting in front of the TV or the computer sounds a lot better than going to practice. Nine times out of ten, they'll feel much better after practice than before. Even as a professional triathlete, I have many mornings when I don't want to get out of bed and many evenings when I don't want to go for a run. The hardest part is just getting out the door.

5. **The Unmotivated**

Some kids just seem to be completely unmotivated when it comes to participating in sports. They have absolutely no interest in it.

Dealing with the Unmotivated Personality

Participating in sports is still part of the answer. If it's just sports they have no interest in, they still need to participate because staying active is vital for every child. If they seem to be unmotivated in every part of their life, sports offer a unique opportunity to see improvement and to get excited about something. If they start to get excited about an athletic activity, this sense of purpose can carry over into other aspects of life. Your role as a parent is to keep providing the opportunity for them to develop an interest in something.

A pet peeve of mine is a parent who will say, "Well...I don't want to make my child do anything they don't want to do." What?! Run that by me again? So what will you say when they don't want to do their homework? What will you say when they don't want to eat their vegetables or they don't want to take their prescribed antibiotics? What happens if they "just don't feel like" going to school on a given day?

A big part of life is doing things you don't want to do because it's in your best interest. The sooner they learn this lesson, the better off they'll be. Part of motivation and of building real (as imposed to inflated) self-esteem is to have the resiliency to accept and overcome challenges. If you allow a child to back down from every new experience or challenge just because they "don't feel like it," you're doing them a disservice and preventing them from developing coping abilities and skills that will serve them well for a lifetime.

Unmotivated is no excuse for unhealthy.

Physical activity is a health issue. Should you force your child to play a sport they hate? Of course not, as long as they substitute it with something else. There has to be some physical activity. Unmotivated is no excuse for unhealthy.

The Talent/Motivation Quadrant

Now that we've looked at different levels and types of motivation, let's see how combining motivation with talent determines a child's opportunity for success. When it comes to a particular activity, your child will fit into one of the quadrants below based on their aptitude for a particular task/activity and their motivation level:

	Talented	Untalented
Motivated	If they possess a natural talent and a focused motivation, then chances are you've found a great activity for them.	If they are very motivated in a particular sport but aren't good at it, stick with it. With a strong drive to improve, they could soon be much better at it.
	Talented	Untalented
Unmotivated	If they are talented, but lack motivation, you owe it to them to keep them involved, at least for a time. Motivation is a spectrum. In time, with continued success, they may develop the drive needed to bring it to the next level.	If they show no particular talent and no particular interest in a given activity, then move on to something else, provided there is something as physically active that they would rather do.

Challenges of Each Quadrant

Quadrant I kids should be praised for their interest and effort. At the same time, you need to keep watch on their well-being and long-term success. A kid who's a great pitcher and loves playing baseball could find himself on the operating table with shoulder surgery, a victim of "too much too soon."

Quadrant II (motivated, but untalented) are a lot of fun to work with. The talent, skills, and techniques can be developed, especially when the athlete is eager to learn and willing to do whatever it takes to improve. Help your Quadrant II child set intermediate goals so they continue to experience success and aren't completely discouraged when they are bested by the Quadrant III kid.

With Quadrant III kids, you have someone with great talent and potential, but they just aren't willing to put in the time, energy, and effort to develop their skill. These kids will see early success, especially at younger ages when physical development, size, and coordination will win out most every time. In time, the late maturing kid will catch up and surpass them. Continue to provide the opportunity for them to take it to the next level. You never know what it might be that finally tips the scales and allows the Quadrant III kid to realize their potential and take their abilities seriously.

Also, reward systems can be effective at getting a Quadrant III kid to move to the more motivated end of the spectrum. At some point, to make the next step, they'll have to start wanting it on their own. In the meantime, offering some type of reward can be a good intermediate step for them, incentive enough for them to give it a chance and allow them to see the intrinsic benefits of applying themselves to a task.

Quadrant IV kids have no discernable interest and little talent in the given activity. If they have another interest, then pursue that. My mantra remains, however: They've got to do something athletic, whether they like it or not.

Pushing Vs. Pulling

Whether your child is generally motivated or unmotivated, kids are kids and it's important to remember that. At some point, they're going to need a little push. What you don't want to do is pull. When you push your child, you're standing behind them, nudging them in the direction of their goals. On the other hand, when you pull a child, you're standing in front of them, trying to force them toward a goal that's usually yours, not theirs.

Four Reasons to Push Your Child

1. Most kids need to be pushed; they can maintain the momentum once they get started. A push provides guidance, direction, and an initial burst of energy.

2. How did you learn to ride a bike? If you're like most people, your parents taught you first by holding onto the bike with you pedaling, then by running alongside you with a hand on the bike, then finally giving you a big push to get going. You couldn't have gotten going without that initial push. If they just ran alongside you with a hand on the seat, you never would have been riding by yourself. Pushing means that you are eventually letting go.

3. When you provide a push, it means they've chosen the direction, you're just helping them to move along their chosen path. A push will take them farther than they could have gone on their own.

4. In chemistry, an equivalent term is "activation energy." All life forms seek out the lowest energy state. To jump to the next phase, there is activation energy required; the spark that moves the process along. Kids often seek out the path of least resistance. That push is what is needed to regain momentum.

How Hard Should I Push?

Because motivation is personal, you can't want it for someone else. If a coach wants "it" (whatever "it" is) more than the athlete, the athlete

> *When you provide a healthy push, you're pushing your child toward their goals.*

probably won't achieve "it." Similarly, if you want "it" more than your kid, you're setting yourself up for disappointment and setting them up to let you down.

How much to push a child depends on their personality. One time at the dinner table, my mom was once again reiterating to me (the overly motivated, stressed-out, perfectionist type), "Don't worry about it, just relax!" My younger brother interjected, "I know! I have been relaxing." Unfortunately, he was the one receiving the message that I needed. John (slow to warm up motivation personality) needed a bigger push to get started. Some pushing is good, and some kids need more of a push than others.

You won't always need to push.

At some point, your child will experience a "conversion." Though typically used in context of a religious awakening, conversions do not necessarily have anything to do with religion. In his epic theological work *Varieties of Religious Experience*, William James defines conversion as when "ideas, previously peripheral in [one's] consciousness, now take a central place, and... form the habitual centre of [one's] energy." So, in order for a conversion to occur, it has to be on the radar screen somewhere. Then something happens, some triggering event, and this idea moves from the periphery of life into the white-hot center.

Often conversions aren't dramatic, but will represent a gradual awakening to a perceived purpose in life. When that point comes, they will have taken ownership over their athletic life. They'll be intrinsically motivated as a result of something that "wakes them up" or triggers a long-term change, and you won't have to push nearly as much.

What you don't want to do is pull.

When you're pushing your child, you're standing behind them; they need the initial momentum and burst of speed to get going. With a push, you're giving them the spark of activation energy, then letting go and allowing them to do it on their own, watching in amazement as they pedal down the road and out of sight.

> *Burnout only happens when someone loses sight of their goals.*

If you're "pulling," this is happening:

1. You're dragging them toward your chosen direction, not theirs. You're taking the lead, depriving them of a chance to learn how to make a good decision.

2. You know you're pulling if you must keep pulling forever—because once you stop pulling, the momentum stops.

When you provide a healthy push, you're pushing your child toward their goals.

One of the parents of a swimmer of mine told me of her husband's early experience in sports. He was an excellent baseball player, but when it came to "his year," the year he would be the starting pitcher on the team and the oldest in the league, he got nervous before the season started and told his parents that he didn't want to play. They didn't make him, and he's never forgiven them for it. Though he's been very successful in life by any measure, he's still convinced that if his parents had just provided the push he needed instead of letting him quit, he'd be finishing up a fifteen-year career in the big leagues!

The best way to determine when and how hard to push your child is to first be clear about what your child's goals are.

A Key Part of Motivation is Having a Good Goal

A good goal is one that's **written** down so it's not forgotten, **specific** so you know exactly what's expected, **challenging** so you don't get bored with it, and **personal** because it means something to you.

Writing a goal down is important. Once words are written down, they take on a new kind of power. You can't forget it even if you want to.

A *specific* goal demonstrates that you know what you want. A goal such as "become a better player" isn't specific enough. Though an admirable aim, it's meaningless unless your child can specify what they mean by "better player." How are they going to measure it? How are they going to know when they get there? When a goal is specific, it has a time frame, and at the end of that time frame, they'll know whether or not they achieved it. Specific doesn't mean that it can't be fluid. If the circumstances change, the goal may change, but it would remain specific.

A *challenging* goal may even be something that seems impossible. Though your child must have smaller intermediate goals to experience some success and maintain motivation, nothing will keep them on track like a challenging goal they care about.

Personal goals are important because it has to mean something to the individual in question. If your child is setting a goal simply because it's what their parents or friends or teachers or coaches want, the chances of ultimate success are minimal.

A good goal provides your child with a map so they know where they'e going.

When my goal was to compete in the Ironman Triathlon at the youngest age allowed, I wrote it down. Because I taped it to the ceiling above my bed, it was the first thing I saw when I got up every morning and the last thing I saw before I went to bed every night. I was visually reminded of my goal at least twice a day.

It was specific. I picked a specific race in a specific year. It doesn't get much more specific than that. I knew I wanted to do the Hawaii

Ironman Triathlon in 1998.

The goal was challenging—make that nearly impossible. When I was twelve, I'd never swam any measurable distance in the ocean, I'd never ridden my bike more than twenty miles or run more than five. However, I was supremely confident that I would be able to do the most difficult one-day endurance event in the world.

The goal was personal. It was something I wanted to do for me, not for anyone else. Good thing, too, because the amount of work and sacrifice I'd endure over the following six years wouldn't have been something I could have done just because someone else wanted me to.

A good goal provides your child with a map so they know where they're going. They may not make huge leaps and bounds toward their goal every day, but if they continue to work toward their goal, their overall progress will be remarkable.

If your child doesn't have a goal and doesn't know what they want, then how will they know when they get it? A goal helps to prevent burnout. Burnout only happens when someone loses sight of their goals. Without a goal, an activity can soon seem meaningless and a child is likely to burn out much more easily.

Once they set their goals, it's up to the child to keep themselves on track. Some people (like a coach, you as a parent, or their teammates) may be able to help them achieve their goals, but at the end of the day, whether they achieve their goals or not depends solely on them, not on other people. Nobody can do it for them. They must take responsibility for the goals they want to achieve. A goal is above all a process, rather than only an end result. Even if they don't achieve exactly what they wanted, it's not a failure. By striving toward something and committing themselves to it, they've learned lessons that will help them with their next goal.

Chapter Summary

Motivation is a complex human emotion, but it boils down to this: In order to motivate someone, they have to first want the result for themselves. The perceived or expected value of the result (the goal) is worth the cost of the sacrifices made to attain the goal. If there's a goal and a desire to achieve it, then you have conditions ripe for a motivated athlete. If there's no goal, there can be no motivation.

Once a goal is established, the challenge becomes keeping your child's focus on their goal. This challenge is different for each child, depending mostly on their level and type of motivation. You know your child better than anyone else. What can you do to help them stay motivated and focused on their goals?

CHAPTER SIX

BALANCE

Joe's Rule #6: "Balance is the forgotten hero of athletic performance."

A slight error in physical balance can have major consequences. You've probably heard of a gymnast whose slip on the balance beam costs her the Olympic Gold, or a skier who couldn't quite negotiate the mogul because he was leaning just slightly the wrong way. But there's a lot more to balance than just the physical aspect of it.

I learned a great lesson about the importance of balance when I was just starting to get serious about cycling. When I was training for the Ironman Hawaii in 1998, I met with a professional cycling coach, Jeff Lockwood. The second time I went to see him, all we talked about was balance. My first thought was, "I'm pretty good at not falling over when I ride, how about showing me how to ride faster?" I soon learned that balance meant a lot more than just not falling over. He showed me how unbalanced I actually was when I was riding; I was making corrections in steering without even noticing it, and it was costing me speed. Working on balance was a way to go faster.

During one of my last training rides before leaving for Hawaii, I was flying down a hill at about 35 mph when my front tire went flat. If I hadn't worked so hard on balance during the previous months, I doubt I could have kept from wiping out. A crash there would have ended any chance I had at the Ironman. Then, on the actual day of the race, the crosswinds coming out of the turn-around town of Hawi hit nearly 40 mph. I was going downhill at 40 mph while fighting off 40 mph crosswinds. A focus on balance, once again, saved me.

Balance is a state of equilibrium where the body is at harmony with its surroundings. It represents the state of optimal functioning in our daily lives. What needs to be balanced when it comes to youth sports? How, as a parent, can you help your child achieve that balance?

How Much is Too Much? How Much is Enough?

Is it possible to have too much of a good thing? Well, food is a "good thing" and we can't live without it. Yet, it's certainly possible to have too much or too little food and there are serious consequences associated with both conditions (obesity and starvation). The healthy approach to food is obviously somewhere in the middle. Too much water is a flood and not enough water is a drought. Too little security led to devastating attacks on our country; too much security leads to grandma getting strip-searched at the airport.

In youth sports, you have overuse injuries and obesity as two ends of the spectrum representing too much activity and not enough activity. Both overuse injuries and childhood obesity are increasing at an alarming rate. The solution is a return to the healthy middle where sports participation is an important part of life, but not an all-consuming obsession. Balance is found in the middle, between the two extremes, for optimal functioning. Too often, people living the problem aren't able to recognize it. Parents need to help their children recognize when things are out of balance, and then assist them in regaining that balance.

Signs that a Child is Out of Balance

There are warning signs at both ends of the spectrum, indicating when a child probably isn't getting enough physical activity and when a child may be doing too much. It's important to be able to recognize these signs so you can help your child regain balance.

Signs of Inactivity

In general, the following signs may indicate that your child isn't getting enough physical activity:

1. If your child isn't getting sixty to ninety minutes of physical activity every day
2. If your child is seriously overweight
3. If your child doesn't know how to "play"
4. If your child is often bored and doesn't know what to "do" if playing video games or watching TV is not an option
5. If your child has the desire to spend all their free time in sedentary activities

Red Flags That Indicate "Too Much"

It's critical to get a sense of whether a sport is controlling your child and your child's life instead of the other way around. If they feel a loss of control and perspective, one activity is playing too large a role in their life and action must be taken. Consider the flowing indicators to be "red flags" that need immediate attention.

1. A drastic and sustained departure from the norm (in their attitude and/or behavior)
2. Prolonged and excessive fatigue
3. Chronic illness and/or injury
4. Rapidly declining grades
5. Feelings of depression
6. Noticeable weight loss or gain

Yellow Flags That May Indicate "Too Much"

The most important thing to watch for when assessing the "yellow flags" is an overall pattern and/or meaningful trends. A single day of reluctance to go to practice or a rough week of training rarely signals a true imbalance. Consider the following indicators to be "yellow flags" that need your attention, but don't *always* mean your child is doing too much.

1. **It's a fight to get them to go to practice or a game.**

   If this is the case, do you also have to fight to get them out the door to school or to sit down and do homework? Is it simply a question of motivation? Consider again what motivates your child and how to keep them focused on their goals.

   Does reluctance to go to practice coincide with a big game approaching or a previous confrontation with the coach? They may be nervous or scared before a big game or they may be hesitant about interacting with their coach again. Find out why your child is reluctant so you can help them deal with whatever is making them nervous.

   Communicate with your child. Ask your child why they don't want to go to practice or a game so you can help them deal with the problem.

2. **Sudden disinterest in their sport.**

   Usually, there's a trigger to a problem. Rarely does a child suddenly lose interest in an activity they previously enjoyed. Is it a new season? If they've been away from the sport for a while, make sure they recognize that it may take some time to regain their rhythm. Have they skipped a season or are they coming back from a prolonged injury or illness? They may be discouraged because something that used to be easy is hard again. They also may be struggling to play at an equal level to friends they used to surpass. Are they prepared for going back to the sport both mentally and physically?

3. **They seem "obsessed" leading up to a big game or competition.**

   When there's a major competition coming up, it's natural to become unbalanced for a little while. If they've invested a great deal of time, effort, and energy preparing for the "big game," it's OK for it to take on major importance and for some other aspects of life to get put on hold. Once the moment of truth passes, it's important to then step back, take some time off, and regain the equilibrium. Think about how a politician running for election has to have a single focus as the big day approaches. This intensity cannot be sustained infinitely. Fortunately, election day comes and goes and some semblance of balance and normalcy returns, win or lose.

> *Burnout is an overused term that's sometimes more of an excuse than an explanation.*

4. **They say they're "burned out."**
    Burnout is an overused term that's sometimes more of an excuse than an explanation. Physical burnout is rare, mental burnout is much more common. Burnout only occurs when the level of commitment is not commensurate with one's goals.

    Physical burnout will occur when demands of a sport exceed a child's physiological limit. It's either a case of too much too young, or too much too soon. Physical burnout can happen even when the spirit is willing, when they want to be out there training, but the body is just too broken down to comply.

    Mental burnout can occur even with the mildest commitment if there's no goal, no perceived reason to partake in the activity, and the grind appears to have no end in sight. To prevent burnout, make sure your child has goals in the activity and that they take some sense of ownership in their participation.

5. **They have a consistently bad attitude before, during, and after practice or a game—and this is out of character for them.**
    The first thing to do is to get to the bottom of what's going on with your child. Is it just a phase they're going through, or is it a symptom of a fundamental imbalance? Did this problem with their sport happen when they made a jump to the next level? If so, then maybe they weren't

prepared for it, either physically or mentally. Something that used to be easy for them is now hard again. They used to be the best on the team, now they're actually getting some time on the bench.

If over-commitment seems to be the problem, you may want to look into scaling back participation level in a given sport. That might mean having to find a different coach or a different team. If over-commitment is the problem, something needs to give. Just make sure, if it's some part of their sports participation that needs to give, they're still getting enough physical activity.

Helping Your Child Regain Balance

In cycling, when a rider crashes, it's usually the result of an overcorrection. If they overlap wheels with another rider and the wheels touch on the right side, physics say they should fall to the right. Instead, most crashes occur to the opposite side. Balance is lost when the wheels touch, but it's the overcorrection that causes the fall. Similarly, when life starts to lose balance, the reaction may be to jerk way too hard in the other direction and compound the problem.

For example, the proper response to an over-commitment is not to withdraw entirely. If your child feels "burned out" and wants to drop an activity completely, letting them do so may be trading one problem for another. The first option would be to scale back participation and reassess their goals. If it's an activity they enjoyed in the past, help them take a step back and regain the balance, rather than letting them throw themselves off balance in another direction.

To prevent burnout, make sure your child has goals in the activity and that they take some sense of ownership in their participation.

Balance is a lot easier to maintain than to regain. The surest way to cure a problem is to prevent it in the first place. At the start of any sports season, begin with clear goals and objectives. This will be simple for a recreational basketball league that has one practice and one game a week and more difficult for a travel soccer team that has four practices a week and tournaments almost every weekend. Be realistic about how your child's life is going to look during the season.

Begin with clear goals and objectives.

Plan some down time. Time to just kick back and relax is important to put into the schedule. Make sure that at younger ages, participation in sports is something that contributes to a well-rounded person, not something all-consuming.

Balancing School and Sports

One of the more difficult things to balance is school and sports. Though challenging, this is far from impossible.

One of the complaints I hear most from parents is how difficult it is for their kids to balance after school activities with homework. The perception is that kids are encumbered with more homework than ever before because schools "teach to the test" during class, then assign the work they're really supposed to be learning to be done at home. While there may be some truth to that, kids are still watching an average of twenty hours of television a week, so perhaps the problem isn't a lack of time, but rather ineffectively prioritizing the time they do have.

In order to balance school and sports, certain ground rules must be laid down. School must come first, and by the time your child has a significant amount of homework, they should have learned how to manage their time. When I was growing up, we were never allowed to watch television or play video games during the week. It was simple; there was no rushing through homework to be done before a favorite show came on. We didn't even consider missing practice to play video games because the option was just never there.

The best way to help your child balance school and sports is to never let them get behind in school. The work isn't overwhelming on a daily basis. The problems begin when it gets put off and allowed to pile up.

Balance and Specialization

School must come first, and by the time your child has a significant amount of homework, they should have learned how to manage their time.

In my conversations with the esteemed John Fowlie, a swim coach at the Australian Institute for Sport, he related to me the importance for balance in life even with the elite level athletes he works with. The AIS (the equivalent of the US Olympic Training Center) forces its athletes to have activities outside of the pool. No swimmer can live onsite unless they also attend school or have a part-time job. If swimming is all they do and there is no balance in the athlete's life, they have nothing to take their mind off of the sport. If they have a below average workout, it eats at them throughout the day. If swimming is all there is, then a period of time where nothing is going right in training means that nothing is going right in life. Not a healthy situation for Olympic-level athletes, or anyone else for that matter.

To be elite in something you have to be somewhat unbalanced. You cannot have a "normal" life and be in the top echelon of any competitive activity. Your job when it comes to your kids is to provide them with the balance early on, until they're mature enough to make the decision about what they want to pursue. You also want them to have enough time to just be a kid. The first priority needs to be health (physical, mental, spiritual), because without health they have nothing.

If, in high school, there's one activity that your child truly wants to be the best at, then you'll have to make the commitment to specialize, and it will have to take priority over pretty much everything else. This is appropriate for a high school athlete who has experienced different sports and knows what they want, not for an eight-year-old who's just starting out. In general, specialization should not be encouraged at an early age. Before puberty, while kids are still growing and developing, it isn't healthy to do the same motions over and over again. There's too much of a risk of overuse injuries.

I cringe when I hear of kids who are eight, nine, or ten and doing one sport six days a week. The problem with doing so much of one activity is not only too much of one thing, but also not enough of anything else. Even if they're good at a sport at a young age, it's hardly an indication of eventual success. Before puberty, you really don't know what the future will bring, so kids need to have a lot of irons in the fire to give them options for the future.

Being involved in a wide range of extracurricular activities increases their exposure to different activities and gives them a greater chance to find something they really love. In order for someone to truly be great, it will eventually have to become their focus; in the meantime, your job is to keep them involved in things until they pick something that will become a focus for them. Everyone needs something to be excited about. It doesn't have to be athletically related at all, but they need something to be passionate about, something that they excel at that sets them apart from everyone else. Give them time, and they will find it. Remember, every child has a genius.

To be elite in something you have to be somewhat unbalanced.

Chapter Summary

Even the most specialized and elite athletes need to maintain balance in their lives. Without it, they tend to lose perspective and can eventually hinder their own performance. The risks of childhood imbalance are even greater. As a parent, it's your job to notice the warning signs that indicate your child may be doing too much or too little. If you find that there's a lack of balance, remember not to over-correct with an equally unbalanced response. The best way to avoid imbalance in the first place is to set goals with your child and keep those goals in mind at all times.

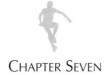

CHAPTER SEVEN

COMPETITION

Joe's Rule #7: "Encourage healthy competition."

There seems to be a tremendous imbalance when it comes to competition in youth sports. A small, but growing number of kids are competing too seriously at too young of an age, and most kids aren't competing enough. Competition is the means by which we improve. By striving together, we push each other to better performances and accomplish more than we could have individually.

Often, major breakthroughs in sports are the result of people competing against each other to be the best or to do something first. Many know Roger Bannister as the man who first broke the four-minute mile barrier in running. He accomplished something that many thought exceeded the limit of human potential. How long did his world record last? A mere forty-six days. John Landy, of Australia, ran 3:58, while being pushed by another competitor the same day—Chris Chataway, who ran 4:04. Would we have landed on the moon if we hadn't been competing with the Soviet Union? We haven't been to the moon since 1972, not because the technology doesn't exist, but because we no longer have the motivation that comes from competition. Competition can bring out the best in people by giving them an incentive to perform at their peak.

Competition isn't the end in itself, but rather a means to an end. It allows us to see the high water mark of human potential by matching up people with similar strengths to strive together toward a noble goal. The problem arises when competition is seen as the end, rather than the means to the end. When "healthy competition" becomes "win at all costs," the innate value of competition is lost. When the focus on results comes too soon, there isn't the foundation to sustain and improve on those results. A focus on winning should only come once the foundation of talent, technique, and condition is in place. As a coach, I don't require the new kids on my team to go to a swim meet if they don't want to. However, I continue to encourage them to try it. Oftentimes, a swimmer will tell me they don't want to compete, but when they finally decide to go to a meet, they realize there's nothing to be afraid of and really enjoy the experience. In team sports, competition is mandatory. You don't sign your child up for soccer and then let them stay home on game day.

The problem with focusing on results too early is that the foundation is not laid for future success. Results may be what you're striving for, but you often don't have direct control over the results. You can't control how well the other team is going to play or how fast another person is going to run; you can only control your own performance. Instead of focusing on results (i.e., telling a six-year-old how important it is to win a game), children should be encouraged to build the foundation for results.

If you've ever wondered why your child isn't winning, think about the process outlined below. Do they have the foundation for success? Chances are they don't!

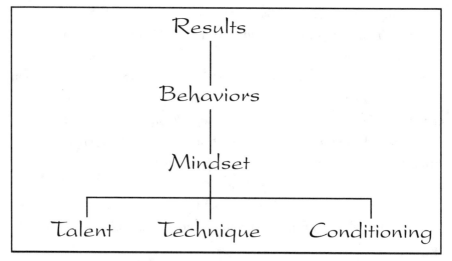

Foundation for Results

The concept of the foundation for results was developed by my good friend Blair Singer. I've modified it to relate to the development of an athlete. The foundation for results consists of three factors: talent, technique, and conditioning. These factors influence the mindset/attitude of the athlete. The mindset, in turn, affects the behaviors, and behaviors lead to results.

Talent

Talent, when it comes to sports, is the innate ability to play a game. Each person has different talents, some evident very young. A child can have a particular aptitude for a sport; they may be able to anticipate plays, master complex motor skills, and generally outperform their peers who practice the same amount as they do. Talent is somewhat unrelated to how much a kid plays a certain sport; rather, raw talent is a certain natural ability that comes much more easily to some than it does to others.

Technique

Technique is what allows someone to further develop talent, and it continues to build a foundation for the game. Technique is a form of conditioning for talent and should be the main focus of youth sports. Proper technique is vital to injury prevention and furthering skill development. At younger ages, many sports favor kids who are bigger and stronger than others. At younger ages, you can "get away" with poor technique if you have the talent and size to overwhelm your opponent. A pitcher may not have good mechanics, but if he's stronger than his opponents, he can still strike them out. However, if technique is poor, it can lead to injuries and stymie future improvement.

Conditioning

Repetition is the key to discovery. Conditioning is the repetition necessary to perform a certain task at a higher level. The more you do a given task, the easier it is to see ways to improve upon it. In sports, conditioning also refers to the aerobic aspect of sports, the stamina necessary to persevere in a

> *The focus should be on what you can control—factors like talent (choosing a sport they have some interest in and aptitude for), technique, and conditioning.*

contest. Conditioning also builds confidence. An athlete can be reasonably confident of their ability to make an important free throw at the end of the game if they've conditioned themselves to hit the shot from fifteen feet away, even when they're tired.

Mindset

Talent, technique, and conditioning combine to form the mindset or the attitude of an athlete. The mindset is of crucial importance. Among top level athletes, the skills, background, and training are pretty much the same. What makes an athlete win is found in the mental phase of the game. If (consciously or unconsciously) someone knows that they have the talent, have worked on technique, and have been faithful with their conditioning, it leads to a positive, confident attitude and a winner's mindset.

The winner's mindset is one of confidence and focus. Athletes with this mindset know that they're up to the challenge because their talent, technique, and conditioning are in line with their goals. Mental strength is a distinct skill set. It's something that needs to be practiced just as physical skills are practiced.

If someone is suffering from a crisis in confidence or a poor mental attitude, it's usually because there's a weakness in their foundation. Either they're convinced that their competitors have more talent ("they are bigger/stronger/faster than me"), they aren't sure of their *technique* ("I just can't make that shot" or "I always swing too late"), or they're uncomfortable with their *conditioning* because they know they haven't put in the time necessary to be successful.

If an athlete is confident in their abilities in each of the three components, it leads to a positive attitude and a winner's mindset. The mindset, in turn, determines the behaviors.

Behaviors

The winner's behaviors can be observed in practices and in games. These are the athletes who continue to work on the talent, technique, and conditioning that form the foundation of a sport. The mindset of confidence and focus builds on itself. The athlete has the focus to work on the behaviors that need improvement. This eventual improvement leads to more confidence. They do the little things necessary to have success. They form good habits in practice, which carry over to games. The good behaviors, both physical and mental, bring about positive results. These positive results reinforce the behaviors and keep the athlete moving along the right track.

Results

Winning results are not the same as winning every game or winning every race. Even the best athletes get upset with their performance, and the best teams sometimes lose games. Often, very little separates the winners from the rest of the field. In baseball, the difference between Hall of Fame numbers (a .333 batting average) and an "average" batting average of .250 is only one additional hit every ten at-bats. Lance Armstrong's win in the 2000 Tour de France was considered a blowout when he won by six minutes. But six minutes over the course of a ninety-two-hour race represents only about .01 percent of the race time.

For young athletes, you must build bottom up. The focus should be on what you can control—factors like talent (choosing a sport they have some interest in and aptitude for), technique, and conditioning. When you put your energy into developing those three factors, the rest falls into place. The results will come in their own time as long as you don't try to force them.

Two Extreme Attitudes Toward Competition

There seem to be two prevalent attitudes toward competition in youth sports today. One focuses too much on the results, ignoring the importance of the foundation necessary for results. The other doesn't focus enough on results, which in many ways also ignores the importance of talent, technique, and conditioning.

Assume that your child will never earn one dime from athletics. How would that affect what they're doing now?

"Win at all costs!"

Parents and coaches who believe in the "win at all costs" mentality are the ones who want to force the results. These are the parents who want to know why there isn't a state championship tournament for their five-year-old's T-ball team. You read stories about parents getting arrested for assaulting each other in the stands of supposedly recreational games, and you hear about the coach who bribed a nine-year-old on his team to injure a mentally disabled teammate so the coach wouldn't have to play the weaker child in the game. This type of competition is obviously unhealthy for children because an early, exclusive focus on results ignores the behaviors, skills, and conditioning that lead to success later on.

If you happen to be one of these parents, imagine, just for the sake of argument, that your child had absolutely zero chance of getting a college scholarship, playing professionally, or competing in the Olympics. Assume that they'll never earn one dime from athletics. How would that affect what they're doing now? *Ideally, it shouldn't affect it at all.* Instead of focusing on remote possibilities and tangible rewards, focus on the healthy aspects of the sport and accentuate the tremendous positives found in sports.

"Competition is bad!"

On the other end of the spectrum are the people who think that "competition" is a four-letter word. They believe this evil thing called competition may make some kids feel bad about themselves and that everyone should win all the time.

In a summer swim league I used to be a part of, there was one group of parents who wanted to score every meet and seemed to try to turn every meet into the Olympics. On the other hand, another group of parents wanted everyone to get a blue ribbon for each event. What's missing from the equation is the balance between these two extremes.

A soccer league in Massachusetts prohibits all soccer teams from keeping score until kids are twelve years old. That's just insulting kids' intelligence; they can count. By that age, they know how many goals each team scored and they know who won and who lost—whether the score is officially kept or not. Extremes like this do a disservice to kids because it suggests to them that results don't matter at all. We worry about damaging a child's self-esteem, so we tell them how perfect they are all the time, robbing them of a sense of accomplishment when they actually achieve something worthwhile.

A study by Jean Twenge of San Diego State University examined the responses of over sixteen thousand college students over a period of twenty-four years (Jean M. Twenge, Ph.D., *Generation Me*, New York: Free Press, 2006). In 2006, over two-thirds of college students had scores above the twenty-year norm for the Narcissistic Personality Inventory. The high expectations these students had for themselves were problematic because they often clashed with reality, resulting in disappointment, depression, anxiety, and loneliness.

We worry about damaging a child's self-esteem, so we tell them how perfect they are all the time, robbing them of a sense of accomplishment when they actually achieve something worthwhile.

Not enough of today's children are being exposed to healthy competition; they're not experiencing the reality that sometimes you win, and sometimes you lose. Because of some intensely negative feelings toward competition and a reaction against certain segments of the population pushing "championship" events for six-year-olds, another segment seems equally passionate about postponing competition until high school. The attack on middle school sports in some places around the country deprives kids of the chance to have a "trial run" at school sports before entering high school.

The middle school district where I grew up eliminated their sports program. It wasn't due to budgetary reasons, like so many other districts, but rather a decision rooted in "philosophy." They were worried about the self-esteem of the kids who got cut from the team. Well, now there's a great solution! Because some kids will "feel bad" if they don't make the team, let's not let anybody play. Other schools require that there be no cuts, and they don't make an "a" team and a "b" team because kids on the "b" team will feel bad. If kids are playing at two different levels, why not create two teams, much like a varsity and a junior varsity team?

It's no fun to be cut. It's happened to me plenty of times. But being cut can open up opportunities in other sports. If it's a sport that your child truly doesn't have the potential to be very good at, it gives them the opportunity to find another sport. If it's a sport that your child really cares about, then the love of the sport will overwhelm the disappointment at being cut and you can find a team or a league where they can continue to play.

How Soon is Too Soon to Compete?

While many kids aren't exposed enough to competition, some kids are pushed into serious competition too young. How soon is too soon to compete? It depends on the kid. Notice how they interact at home. How do they handle the "competitive" aspect of board games or cards? Can they handle winning and losing so they don't see their self-worth determined by an external result? In my experience, most kids are ready for competition at age five or six. This means they have an understanding of what it means to be part of a team and can begin to learn the rules of a game.

More "competitive" leagues shouldn't start much earlier than nine or ten. Still, know your child. If they're in a more competitive league, monitor their progress and demeanor. If it's too much for them, then back off. There's nothing to be gained and much to lose by forcing a child to compete at a level they're uncomfortable with at an age when they can't handle it.

Whatever you do, please don't buy into the notion that if your child isn't on the traveling team at age eight, they'll never make the high school team/college team/professional leagues. Some youth football leagues start kids as young as seven in tackle football with full pads. They're led to believe unless you're serious and make a major commitment in grade school, you can never amount to anything in the sport. There are plenty of stories of athletes who got a relatively late start in their sport and went on to achieve at the highest level.

Effort And Results

It's important to help your child understand the difference between effort and results. Sometimes, we get great results with little effort. Other times, we can get disappointing results with tremendous effort. One reason why timed sports are so healthy is that kids can compete against themselves. In a sport like running or swimming, a child can see their improvement. If they ran a mile in 8:15 and got third place, and in the next competition they ran 8:05 and got sixth place, they're getting better, not worse. As long as they're competing against their previous performances, they can have a sense of accomplishment that's independent of how other people perform, which is something that they have no control over. Healthy competition comes from focusing on a child's efforts and how those efforts are connected to their individual results.

I had a parent tell me that her child was disappointed because he didn't make the "finals," a special day of competition for the top eight swimmers in each event. They had a talk at the end of the season about why it was important to the child to make the top eight and what he thought he could do to earn that distinction the following year. The next year, he made the top eight in two events and achieved a goal he had set for himself. What really matters in this story? Will anyone really care a year from now what place they got in a meet? Probably not. What matters is the process. He didn't make it one year, decided that's what he wanted to do the next year, and then did what was necessary to achieve the goal. Here's the best part: In the beginning of the next school year, he got a 3/10 and 4/10 on his first two spelling tests. Not quite up to anyone's expectations. His mother took the opportunity to ask him, "What grades do you want to get on these tests?" He answered, "A nine or ten." Then his mother said, "Let's set a goal, just like you did with swimming. What do you need to do to get those results?" They made a list of how he should study for the upcoming tests. The results? A 9/10 and then a 10/10.

The Curse of Early Success

At some point (starting around age eleven), kids who are used to winning everything see their initial advantage evaporate. The United States Swimming National Age-Group Records provide an interesting case study in youth development. If someone familiar with competitive swimming looked at the 10 & Under records, they wouldn't recognize any of the names because hardly any of the kids who hold those records went on to major success later. Less than 5 percent of the kids ranked in the top one hundred of all time in the 10 & Under age-group were on the same list for the seventeen- to eighteen-year-old age-group. The records for eleven- to twelve-year-olds include some of the names of kids who later when on to Olympic glory. By the time you hit the thirteen- to sixteen-year-old records, pretty much every name on the list is one that's a household name in the swimming community.

Early success in a sport is a blessing or curse depending on the personality of your child. For some, an early taste of success will drive them to work even harder to continue to improve. Too often, it's a curse, which left untreated, will hinder their development as an athlete. Jim Collins, in his book *Good to Great*, says: "The Good is the enemy of great..." People become satisfied with a certain level of success and are unwilling or unable to demand more of themselves to reach toward the limits of their potential.

When a child experiences early success in sports, they get used to winning without having to do the work. Because of their innate physical and talent advantage, they're far ahead of their peers and able to win consistently. The key is what happens

If a child has never struggled, they don't have the coping strategies to deal with setbacks.

as the child ages. As everyone else develops and this early edge is lost, the child must now work for the success. They'll eventually meet up with another athlete who had to compensate for a lack of skill early on by increasing their effort. This other child will have learned the discipline necessary to be successful at the next level.

One of my friends, a professional ski instructor, was asked to train a ten-year-old girl. She had entered a local race and finished second place with no training. The mother was excited about her daughter's new sport and wanted to capture this enthusiasm because she had rarely shown an interest in competitive sports. The girl competed in several local races and consistently placed at the top. Barely a year after her first local race, she went to a regional race. She did really well and placed second in a field of thirty kids, but she cried on the way home and soon after quit skiing. In her mind, she had spent a lot of time practicing, but her results didn't improve. She placed second in a small local race with no practice and couldn't comprehend that second place in a regional competition represented significant improvement.

This a perfect example of the curse of early success. Had she finished fifth or tenth in her first race and enjoyed it, her faithful practice would have resulted in tangible improvement. Because she had done so well right away,

In our current "instant gratification" culture, kids are expecting to see results immediately and without much effort.

there was nowhere to go but down. She apparently only liked skiing because she was good at it. She didn't like practicing, she liked winning. She had unreasonable expectations for herself and when she was unable to immediately reach those expectations, she quit.

The same problem is seen in the academic world with the transition from high school to college. Some kids who were straight "A" students in high school find themselves flunking out of college. Academics came easily to them in high school, so they didn't have to learn the study skills and time management habits that are necessary for success. They were naturally smart enough to get by without needing them. However, in college, when the academic workload takes a quantum leap, they find that their natural smarts aren't enough to cut it anymore. Because they've never struggled, they don't have the coping strategies to deal with setbacks and may lack the study skills necessary to pull themselves out of a hole. They aren't used to having to deal with failure and may convince themselves to drop out altogether.

This same situation happens in sports. How many of you have a child who wants to win and be successful, but is unwilling to do the work necessary? If they were at first ahead of the rest of their peers, but now have to work a lot harder just to experience the same level of success, what will keep them motivated? The answer is: "A goal." They have to want something within the perimeters of the sport for themselves. It can't be something that the parent wants for them or they'll just be doing it to get some external award. "Break that record, and I'll get you a puppy," doesn't work for long. It has to be something they want for themselves and want badly enough that they'll consistently stick with it through the ups and downs.

Improvement and Consistency

The key to improvement is consistency. Professional baseball players take hundreds of pitches in batting practice, even though they've been playing the game for years. Pro basketball players may shoot hundreds of free throws at a stretch so they feel comfortable at the line when the balance of the game hangs on one free throw. By doing something over and over and over, the action becomes second nature. When a person has a truly refined skill, they can feel the tiniest difference in technique and see what effect it has on performance. Only when a person has swung a bat thousands of times does the action become so ingrained that the smallest difference is noticeable.

In our current "instant gratification" culture, kids are expecting to see results immediately and without much effort. Many want the success that comes with achievement, but are unwilling to put in the work necessary to be successful. Approached the right way, at the right age, sports can help teach kids the value of working hard in order to improve results as they reach toward a goal.

Competition and Goals

When I speak to school groups, I tell them about two of my previous goals. The Ironman Hawaii is widely considered to be the toughest one-day endurance event in the world. Each year, nearly fifty thousand people attempt to qualify for Ironman, but the field is limited to around fifteen hundred. To qualify, you have to place at the top of your age-group at one of these Ironman qualifying events. The youngest age-group is eighteen- to twenty-four-year-olds. So having just turned eighteen, I would have to beat the best twenty-four-year-olds in the world just to make it to the starting line. A challenging goal, indeed!

As 1998 approached, my goal was no longer to simply finish the Ironman, but to finish it in less than ten hours. No person eighteen years old had ever done that. My goal even evolved the week before the race when I realized that the Ironman record for the 19 & Under age-group was 9:59.04. I decided that as long as I was going to break the ten-hour barrier, I may as well go another minute or so faster and pick up the record in the process! The competition I had set up within myself to break ten hours ended with a finish time of 9:57.10.

Ironman is the most significant goal that I've had, but far from the only one. I have set many, many goals...some I achieve, some I don't. I think back to what would have happened had I not qualified for the Ironman, or if I had failed to finish. Does that mean that everything I worked for would have been for nothing? Absolutely not! Even if I had failed to finish the race, the process of having the goal, of having something great to work toward would have been worth it. Though my Ironman goal was a success any way you look at it, I have had other major goals that didn't work out the same way.

My senior year in college was unlike any other year I ever experienced. I kept thinking that at some point life would slow down enough for me to take a breath, but that was not to be. Not only did I have a senior thesis to develop, I also had to make good on my goal of becoming a Rhodes Scholar. Before I entered college, I made my goal to win the Rhodes Scholarship. The Rhodes Scholarship is the world's most prestigious post-graduate scholarship and also the most difficult to win. It's awarded to the top college graduates from all over the world. There are thirty-two Rhodes Scholarships given each year in the United States and usually around a thousand applications. The standards just to apply are pretty daunting. It's said not to bother applying unless your GPA is above 3.8 and you have substantial achievement in the fields of academics, athletics, and community service.

Take the opportunity to point out examples of failure leading to success to your child; the stories are all around you.

I had built up a solid undergraduate record and was ready for the challenge. At the end of my freshman year, I went to see the dean in charge of the applications and he asked me what my GPA was. I told him a 3.91. His response was, "I guess that's OK, but don't let it drop any lower." I took it as a challenge and received a 4.0 for all of my remaining classes over the next three years. That gave me a 3.96, which qualified me for the Rhodes. I recruited the aid of Professor

Janet McCracken to write my personal statement, and it took seventeen tries before Janet and I were happy with the essay and countless more hours to condense my list of activities in college to the requisite two pages. I spent well over a hundred hours preparing this application. Not to mention four years with this goal in mind, making decisions such as which classes to take and what to do in my unscheduled time in order to give myself the best possible chance at success.

I was thrilled to hear that I made the cut for an interview and flew back to Arizona with visions of two years at Oxford dancing in my head. I performed well in the interview, but didn't make the next cut and came back to school with nothing. It was strange to see a four-year goal end so abruptly, but like the Ironman goal, the success wasn't in the destination, but rather the journey. The challenges that the Rhodes endeavor presented kept me motivated and on track during college. Even though the result didn't match my expectations, it was worth the effort and certainly wasn't a waste of time. Just as the Ironman goal gave me something to pursue during the major life changes of junior high and high school, the Rhodes goal kept me focused on what was important during my four years at Lake Forest College.

In the traditional sense, one of my goals was an astonishing success and the other a spectacular failure. If one were only to judge the success of the goal based strictly on the final results, then the descriptions would be that simple. The Ironman goal was an unqualified success. In six short years, I went from just another kid to one of the top young endurance athletes in the world. I accomplished what seemed impossible, and I accomplished it in record time. The Rhodes goal would appear to be a spectacular failure. I invested hundreds of hours in a process that didn't give me the desired result. There was no consolation prize, no parting gift for making it as far as I did in the Rhodes application process. Only a "yes" or a "no"—and I got a "no." This, however, didn't make me a failure. It wasn't about what I wanted to have or what I wanted to do, but who I wanted to be. The person I became in the process was worth the investment. Take the opportunity to point out examples of failure leading to success to your child; the stories are all around you. You've probably lived some of them.

The Value of Competition

Both of my goals were very competitive in nature. The competition I experienced drove me to accomplish more than I could have on my own. It also provided the opportunity for me to experience what it felt like to win and the opportunity for me to deal with the experience of losing.

Competition gives you the opportunity to win.

Winning is fun! Properly structured, competition allows those with a combination of talent, motivation, and skill a chance to shine among their peers. This success can fuel the drive to continue to improve in order to continue to experience this success.

Competition gives you the opportunity to lose and learn from it.

Learning to lose is just as important as learning to win. Most kids who say, "I don't like to compete" really mean, "I don't like to lose." Learning how to lose and learning how to fail and persevere are important skills that matter in real life. You can't win all the time. I know that. You know that. Kids need to learn that there's no shame in losing or falling short of expectations if they put forth à full effort. They need to know how to learn from failure and move on. If a child continues to work on the foundation of talent, technique, and conditioning, the results will come in time.

Competition pushes you to achieve more than you're likely to on your own.

As the Ironman and Rhodes stories illustrate, I wouldn't have been able to achieve what I did without the push from my competitors. Even though I didn't know who they were at the time, I knew that the Ironman was a very difficult race to qualify for and the Rhodes was a very difficult scholarship to win because of the competitors I was up against.

Chapter Summary

An early, exclusive focus on results ignores the underlying process that leads to results. Focus on talent, technique, and conditioning. These three factors influence the mindset of an athlete, which influences behaviors, which in turn lead to results. Competition is very healthy; it's the "win at all costs" mentality that's unhealthy.

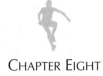

CHAPTER EIGHT

ACCENTUATE THE POSITIVE

Joe's Rule #8: "Help your child build character through participation in sports."

Sports present the opportunity to have clear, measurable goals. But a goal is far more than a specific achievement. A goal is a vision for the future. It's not about what your child wants to have, and it's not about what they want to do. It's about who they want to BE. The true value of a life-changing goal is not what someone does to get there, but rather who they become in the process.

Sure, you'd like your child to be successful in sports, but you probably care more about the person they're becoming than the games they win, the trophies they collect, or the records they break. Don't lose sight of that. It's possible to have results and achievement without success, just as it's possible to have success without results or achievement. The world is full of "successful" people who have achieved a lot, but the person they became in the process is not necessarily what you would want for your child.

Let's take a look at the ways participation in sports provides the opportunity for character development and how you can accentuate the positives for your child.

Sportsmanship

Sportsmanship can be defined as winning with class, losing with grace, always giving one's best, and never giving up. The more experience a child has in sports, the more they're able to put a given contest in perspective. Though

> *A goal is a vision for the future. It's not about what your child wants to have, and it's not about what they want to do. It's about who they want to BE.*

some games or events take on immense importance, someone with enough experience knows that, win or lose, the sun does indeed come up the next day and life will go on. Let's look at the description of sportsmanship more closely...

Winning with class/Losing with grace

A true sportsman can take winning and losing in stride. It's normal, and certainly OK, to be thrilled with a win and distraught with a loss. The more you invest in an undertaking, the more its result will matter to you. The most important thing to remember is that life goes on. When I coach swimming, what I try to impress most to my swimmers about competition is to take each race one at a time. At a given swim meet, a child might swim five events in a day. It's a great opportunity for them to experience elation or disappointment over and over again within a period of a couple hours.

When I was swimming competitively, starting at the age of seven, I was always taking things far more seriously than anyone else my age. I would get incredibly nervous before a competition and turn each important meet into the biggest event in my life. It took years, but I finally figured out that I'd have some races I was happy with, some I wasn't happy with, and life would keep rolling.

By high school, I mastered the technique of "leaving the swim in the warm down pool." After each swim at a meet, I would "warm down" or swim several hundred yards to flush the lactic acid from my muscles. I would allow myself that set period of time to care about how the meet went. I wouldn't think about it until I walked over and got in the warm down pool. Whether it was a good swim or a bad swim, I would acknowledge the emotion while I was warming down; but as soon as I was done, I would climb out of the pool and leave the swim behind.

Before I used this technique, I would let myself get upset about a swim and then let my negative attitude affect how I swam the rest of the day. If it was a good swim, I still needed to move on and not let the one success cause me to lose focus on the rest of the day's events. Once I got comfortable with this routine, it was easier for me to be able to show grace in defeat and class in victory. Even though I was, and still remain, a very intense person, I've learned how to control and harness my emotions so they don't negatively affect the rest of my life.

Always giving one's best

Sportsmanship isn't just how your child acts or what your child says before or after a game, it's also revealed in how the game is played. Being a good sport means being a team player.

I notice a pattern in some athletes who quit on themselves. If they're swimming a race and find themselves behind, they just give up. They would rather be able to tell themselves, "I didn't really try" than to know that they gave their best effort and still came up short. That's poor sportsmanship and can lead to some bad life habits.

A poor effort is never excusable. I don't have a problem losing to someone who's better than I am, but I can't justify losing to someone who tried harder. Stress to your athlete that it's OK to not be as talented as someone else; what matters is that they always do their personal best.

A clear example of sportsmanship (both good and bad) occurred in Super Bowl XXVII in 1993. The Cowboy's defensive lineman, Leon Lett, picked up a fumble and was about to give Dallas a 59-17 lead when the Bills wide receiver, Don Beebe, chased him down and knocked the ball out of his hands a yard from the goal line as Lett slowed down to showboat. Not only was this a display of poor sportsmanship on the part of Lett, not exactly winning with class as his team was ahead nearly forty points, but great sportsmanship on the part of Beebe. This play was not going to make a difference in the outcome of the game, but he refused to be on the field giving less than a full effort.

Never giving up

Never giving up can mean not giving up on a teammate who's having a rough time or not giving up during a race that's painful. It also means not giving up on yourself. A true sportsman knows that you're not knocked out if you get up. Life presents many challenges, and sports provide a great opportunity to teach your child how to meet those challenges. Sportsmanship means never giving up, tackling challenges, and rising above obstacles.

When I was playing recreational soccer at ages eight and nine, my dad made sportsmanship a high priority for me. After every game I played, he had me find the best player on the opposing team, introduce myself, and personally congratulate him on a good game. He said, "You never know when you'll be on the same team as one of those guys, you want to start building friendships with your opponents now." It wasn't an easy thing to do, especially after a loss. When I was eight, I hated going up to the person who was most instrumental in my team's loss and congratulating him. It was a little bit more fun after a win, but still very awkward at first.

I never thought it would amount to anything. These kids on different teams seemed so far removed from me, and I couldn't imagine playing on their team. Sure enough, when I was nine, a select team was formed from the league that included all the best players on each of the teams. I was suddenly on the same team as all of the kids I had been getting to know after each game, win or lose.

To accentuate this positive: *Keep in mind the goal, the vision for the future, "who they will become." Sports have the ability to draw out certain personality* *characteristics; make sure sportsmanship is one of them. Encourage your child to win with class, lose with grace, always give their best, and never give up.*

Winning and Celebrating Successes

Winning is fun. It's as simple as that. The thrill of victory, the sensation of coming through with a great performance when it matters most, the confidence that grows as your child comes through when the team needs them. Though winning isn't all that matters, it's an important aspect of any sport. Nobody plays a game to lose. Keep in mind that if your child has never lost, then winning doesn't mean anything.

Any child who plays sports for any period of time will have some level of measurable success. Whether that success is meeting a personal goal that only matters to the child or winning a major competition celebrated by everyone isn't really the point. The boundless joy that results from a major personal triumph is something that everyone should be able to experience. Participation in sports offers many opportunities to experience that.

To accentuate this positive: Celebrate success with your child. Let them enjoy the feeling that comes with putting out a full effort in the field of play and emerging victorious. Let them experience what it feels like to set a personal goal and then achieve it.

Role Models and Heroes

In a 2000 study by the Kaiser Family Foundation, 73 percent of children say that "famous athletes" are people they "look up to or want to be like." A hero is someone who's larger than life and can inspire your child through their example. Though the fallen heroes are often the ones who grab the headlines, many athletes are quietly putting in heroic efforts and accomplishing amazing things. Here are two examples of outstanding role models:

In her book, *Swimming to Antarctica*, Lynne Cox describes her childhood experience as an average swimmer; she was someone who tried hard but didn't have a lot of talent. Then she discovered she had an amazing ability for open water swimming and dealing with the challenges of incredibly long distances and extreme conditions. As a teenager, she set the world record for swimming the English Channel and then went on from there, literally swimming her way around the world. She swam some of the most treacherous stretches of ocean, including the Bering Strait, the Strait of Magellan, and the Cape of Good Hope. She even recorded a mile-long swim in Antarctica in thirty-three degree water. Growing up, she didn't have the "swimmer's body" and didn't have the talent other kids had. Rather than giving up, she found her niche and accomplished heroic feats.

Dick and Rick Hoyt are Ironman legends. They've never won the race, but everyone who's competed at the Ironman World Championship knows their names. Rick was born with severe physical handicaps, but high mental function. The doctors said he should be "put away" because there was "no hope of a normal life." Together with his father, they have far exceeded any definition of normal. They compete as a team in many running and cycling events as well as triathlons. They have completed the Ironman with Dick, now sixty years old, pulling his son in a raft behind him during the swim race, riding a custom-made bike for two with Rick on the front during the bike race, and pushing Rick in a wheelchair during the running race.

Rather than looking at the reasons why it couldn't be done, "Team Hoyt" just went ahead and did it. Dick took on this mammoth athletic endeavor when he first entered a race pushing Rick in a wheelchair. Though not at all a distance runner, Dick agreed to push Rick in his wheelchair. They didn't win; in fact they finished next to last, but they did finish. After the race, Rick told his father that he just didn't feel handicapped when they were competing. They've been competing ever since.

To accentuate this positive: Point out heroes when you see them. It's not always the biggest names or the highest-paid stars, but the hero for your child can be the person who inspired them to reach inside and unlock the potential that they couldn't reach before.

Self-Perception

For many people, part of their identity is tied to their activities and what they enjoy doing. Just as art or music may be a substantial part of someone's life, sports offer yet another activity to be passionate about. Sports can help a child to build a positive identity.

Kids who perceive themselves as athletes may be more inclined to make healthy choices outside of the playing field. When I was growing up, I had the Ironman goal to keep me focused. I could evaluate each choice by asking if it would get me closer to my goal or farther away. I avoided many of the "detours" of high school by keeping my goal my priority. I knew what it would take to be an Ironman, what it meant to be a true athlete. Alcohol, cigarettes, and drugs were certainly not part of that definition.

To accentuate this positive: Talk with your child about how they see themselves as an athlete. What does it mean to be an athlete? What role do sports play in their self-perception? What can you do to reinforce a healthy self-perception?

Team Building

A team structure is different from the structure of a family or a class, the two other main social groups that a child is a part of early in life. An ideal team combines a group of peers with similar interests who strive toward a common goal. A good team environment has something to offer every child, but can fill different roles for different individuals. A functioning team has solid leadership from coaches and captains. This team challenges each other in practice, trying to make each other better and eventually more successful in competition against other teams. Successful teams hold each other accountable, but do not dwell on mistakes or belittle an error. Each member knows that next time they could be the one who makes a crucial mistake and needs the rest of the team to be supportive.

There are lessons that children will be able to take away from team situations to prepare them for later in life. Corporate managers often put together "teams" to work on various projects. A sports team can function well or be dysfunctional; a corporate team can have the same characteristics. Teamwork is the division of a team's responsibilities to its members, who are all working toward the same goal. Different people fill different roles on the team, and each role matters. If a child plays center on the basketball team, they'll learn that it doesn't necessarily make them any better than the point guard or the small forward; each person just has a different role to fill.

It's distressing to hear of kids quitting sports because they don't get along with their teammates. It's sad that the team isn't living up to its potential, but it's an obstacle often presented in team sports. The ability to get along with disagreeable people is a valuable skill. At the professional level, coaches have to keep many large egos in check and focus everyone involved on the good of the team. By that stage of the game, most athletes can set aside personal differences. Though professional athletes can usually put aside petty differences, it's often difficult for children to do the same. Learning to work together with a diverse group of people is one of the valuable lessons that can be learned through early participation in sports.

> *To accentuate this positive: Make sure that the team your child joins is a healthy, constructive team. Recognize that no team is perfect and a disagreement with a teammate is a great opportunity to work on conflict resolution.*

Fun

Sports can be a lot of fun. It can be seen in the joy abounding in the exuberance of youth spilling out onto the playing field. Or the joy of athletes lost in a world where time stands still, the rest of the world melts away, and all that matters is putting the ball in the goal one more time. If you talk to any long-term successful athlete, they'll say, nearly without exception, that they're primarily motivated by the love of the sport. The reason that top athletes continue to stay in the game long after they're financially secure is often for the same reason they started the sport in their youth—it's fun. There's intrinsic enjoyment that comes from being active.

To accentuate this positive: Keep in mind that most children are motivated by fun. For many, after the drudgery of a full day of school, they want to do something "fun." Work with your child to find outlets of athletic expression that are fun for them.

Skill Development and Improvement

Kinesthetic learning is often developed in sports. Most sports are easy to learn, but impossible to master. Therein lies the opportunity for continual growth. Take cycling, for example. It's a relatively easy sport to learn. When I worked with the cycling coach I mentioned earlier, he started out by showing me the six different angles your foot should pass through as you complete each pedal stroke, each leg revolving at a rate of ninety times per minute. Then we progressed to how to carry greater speed through turns, how to effectively climb and descend a hill, how to sustain a given pace through varying terrain. All of a sudden I realized how little I actually knew about riding a bike and understood that it was impossible to do it all perfectly. That's why the best athletes in every sport still have coaches.

Michael Jordan, when he was the best basketball player in the world, hired a personal trainer whose only goal was to get Jordan the ability to jump one inch higher. For top athletes, it isn't enough to be "good," they want to be "great." Skill development never ends. It should be of primary importance in any youth sports program. Good technique helps to build the foundation of success for an athlete.

Life is all about learning new things and how to apply them. Some of the same patterns of learning in sports are directly applicable to learning how to master other skills in life. For example, participation in sports teaches you that the more you do a certain task, the more you learn about it, and the more you learn ways to improve upon your past performance. From one game or one practice or one season to the next, there's a learning process that occurs. You can figure out what worked and what didn't work. What will it take to make the leap to the next level? It's similar to a job review at work. What did you do well? How can you improve on your past performance and move from average or "good" to true excellence in your given task?

To accentuate this positive: Stress personal improvement and development. Motivate your child based on improvement and how their performance compares to their previous performances. It's something they can control. "Winning" depends greatly on how other people do. Don't let their evaluation of their personal improvement depend on what other people are doing.

A Healthy Lifestyle and Life Skills

Even the best athletes have to fit sports in with the rest of their life. Being completely dedicated to a sport is a mixed blessing. By definition, pursuing excellence in a specific sport is unhealthy. There isn't a single sport where its top athletes are the picture of a well-rounded, well-adjusted, healthy individual. That's because they don't give away the medals and the prize money for those criteria. It's a meritocracy based strictly on performance. There is certainly nothing wrong with trying to be the best at something. But for every Olympic champion, there are literally hundreds, if not thousands, of athletes who have trained just as hard and sacrificed just as much, but come away empty-handed. That's why winning shouldn't be the only goal. Being "in shape" is much more than looking a certain way or fitting into a given outfit; it's about health and making the right choices and forming good habits early in life to carry into the future.

With my swim team, we have a set of life skills that we work through each season. In a period of eight weeks, we talk about one topic each week. Many of the kids I coach have a lot of talent and will go far in the sport of swimming if they remain dedicated to it. But *all* of the kids I coach have what it takes to be successful in life and become outstanding members of society. Given the choice, I'd rather see a kid grow up to be a healthy, happy, productive adult rather than just someone who can swim really fast.

To accentuate this positive: Maintain perspective. Think about how a certain sport, activity, or experience has the potential to influence the development of your child. Focus on ways to use their activities to emphasize a healthy lifestyle and to develop skills that will serve them well throughout life.

Chapter Summary

Playing sports provides the opportunity to develop character. Simply playing sports doesn't build character. But as a parent, you can shape the experience into one that is positive and life-enhancing for your child. Think about this: The positive moral development from sports in England was so pervasive that the Duke of Wellington claimed, "Victory at Waterloo was won on the playing fields of Eton."

CHAPTER NINE

MINIMIZE THE NEGATIVE

Joe's Rule #9: "Shed light on the shadow of sports."

The Shadow

"(The shadow) is everything in us that is unconscious, repressed, undeveloped and denied. These are dark rejected aspects of our being as well as light, so there is positive undeveloped potential in the Shadow that we don't know about because anything that is unconscious, we don't know about. The Shadow is an archetype. And what an archetype simply means is that it is typical in consciousness for everyone. Everyone has a Shadow. This is not something that one or two people have. We all have a Shadow and a confrontation with the Shadow is essential for self-awareness."

In this somewhat complicated definition, Carl Jung defines a shadow lurking within each person as something that is hidden in the unconscious, buried from view. I interpret it as something dangerous or negative. People are not the only entities to have a shadow. Every positive characteristic of sports has a shadow lurking in the darkness. Within every hero lies a veiled villain, within every positive hides a negative, within every life lurks a death. Sports can lead to a healthy, physically fit lifestyle, or a life ruined by drugs in pursuit of material success. Sports can lead to teamwork or result in a dysfunctional unit with infighting members. Healthy competition can be an outgrowth of sports, but sports can also lead to situations where people put the outcome ahead of all other considerations, regardless of who is harmed in the process. The shadow characteristic lurking behind the light of sports must be recognized.

There are a number of problems that can arise in pursuit of athletics. Instead of ignoring them, the negative aspects need to be addressed so they can be minimized. They can never be eliminated completely, but by working to keep the focus on the positive, the youth sports experience will be better for everyone involved. Each of the following sections talks about one of the shadows of sports. The "ShadowBuster" section addresses how to turn the negative into a positive and offers questions to discuss with your child when the shadowy subject comes up. Depending on your child's age and comprehension level, you may have to tailor the question to fit their level of understanding.

Poor Sportsmanship

Sportsmanship was defined in the previous chapter as winning with class, losing with grace, always giving one's best, and never giving up. Poor sportsmanship is quite the opposite: gloating over a win, throwing a fit over a loss, letting your team down with a poor effort (in practice or in games), and giving up on yourself or your teammates. Poor sports just aren't fun to be around because they take everyone down with them.

Too often, the poor sportsmanship isn't from the kids, but from the parents and coaches. When emotionally engaged, people tend to lose all sense of reason. That's why when under pressure, in a situation where the emotion is high, you can't think of anything to say; yet twenty minutes later when you've cooled off, you're able to think of the perfect response. Because there are few acceptable outlets for emotion in our society, sports have emerged to fill the gap. People can become delirious or despondent based on the results of a game played thousands of miles

There are a number of problems that can arise in pursuit of athletics. Instead of ignoring them, the negative aspects need to be addressed so they can be minimized.

away where "their team" is competing. Put your own kids in the mix and the emotion goes up even more. It comes to the point where you have a large number of "intelligence-impaired," emotional people worked up and putting pressure on an eight-year-old to make a free throw. The shadow of poor sportsmanship is so pervasive, it can't be ignored.

ShadowBuster:
Kids notice how a coach acts and how their parents act. They're great observers. Don't miss an opportunity to display good sportsmanship. Talk about some recent examples of poor sportsmanship, both in professional sports that they've observed and in their own sport that they may have seen at a practice or a game.

ShadowBuster Questions:
• Tell me about a time when you saw someone display poor sportsmanship. Why do you consider it to be poor sportsmanship?

• What should the person have done in that situation to model good sportsmanship?

• What causes people to act inappropriately during a stressful, emotional situation?

• What can you do yourself when faced with a similar situation?

• Who is someone on your team that you think of as a model of good sportsmanship? Why? What do they do that other people don't do?

• What are three things you can do in the next week to model good sportsmanship for your teammates?

Over-Emphasis on Results: "Win at All Costs"

We're a results-driven culture. That's a good thing, because in the "real world" results matter. But until a child has the skills necessary to produce the results, the efforts will be futile. Until the processes are developed, an over-emphasis on results will impede progress. Child athletes are not "miniature adult" athletes. Their cognitive abilities are different, their motivations may be different, and their life experiences are vastly different.

The problem with too much of a focus on results is that the physical characteristics that allow a child to be successful at a young age do not directly translate into success later. As I've already mentioned, if a child can pair good coordination with their size, they can become unstoppable. Most youth sport leagues have age "cutoff" days. A kid fortunate enough to have a birthday just after the cutoff date enjoys the advantage of being older than the competition. In high school, a single year of age may not make a huge amount of difference, but there are major developmental (both cognitive and physical) differences between a seven-year-old and an eight-year-old. Someone unlucky enough to just miss the age cutoff faces an uphill battle, always having to compete against older kids.

Again, a healthy balance must be struck between the opposite ends of the spectrum. While it's foolish to reward and encourage a team of eight-year-olds solely on the basis of wins and losses, it's equally ridiculous to grant them no competitive outlet. It's possible to have good, healthy competition, yet not make winning the only goal. When winning becomes the only goal, the other parts of sports and the importance of displaying good sportsmanship get lost in the process.

A healthy balance can be seen in the Ironkids Triathlon series. The Ironkids series was, at one point, a national series of races in nineteen cities, culminating with a National Championship. The series was for kids ages seven to fourteen with age-appropriate distances. Though each race recognized the top three boys and girls in each age-group with a medal ceremony, the slogan for the series was, "Every finisher is a winner." The series recognized accomplishment and inspired kids to train hard to win their age-group and even a chance to get an expenses-paid trip for their family to the national championships. But the medalists weren't the focus of the series. Each child's name was announced as they ran under the giant rainbow finish line, breaking the finisher tape. Each finisher also received a finisher's pin.

Ironkids was successful in rewarding and encouraging competition and the pursuit of excellence, but recognized the effort it took from each child to complete the race. They didn't pretend that everyone was the same. They didn't give every child a gold medal. But they did their best to make the race a celebration of youth fitness and rewarded those who completed the race. At each race, they also presented the "Spirit Award" to an entrant who may not have been fast, but who best exemplified the spirit of sportsmanship.

The more a child continues with a certain sport, the more the "win at all costs" mentality will grow; the more a child invests in a sport, the more seriously they'll take the outcome. If they play baseball in the spring just to have something to do, a loss won't matter as much because there's no investment on their part. If they play ball fifty weeks a year and it consumes nearly all of their free time, the important games are going to seem like the only thing that matters.

When I was swimming twenty-five hours per week in high school, I had my "blinders" on the month before a major competition. It was as though my whole life was built around that weekend, and I couldn't even bring myself to think about what life would be like once it was over. This would happen two to three times per year. Because so much of my life was taken up by swimming, these championship meets seemed like they were all that mattered.

ShadowBuster:
Guard against the "win at all costs" mentality by keeping perspective yourself. Kids take their cues from you. If you continually talk about how important it is to win and if you value winning above all else, then don't be surprised when your kid follows suit. Emphasize the process over the results. At younger ages, there are shortcuts to immediate improvement that are detrimental in the long run. If you consistently emphasize the process, the results will eventually be able to speak for themselves.

ShadowBuster Questions:

- How does it feel to win?

- How does it feel to lose?

- What makes losing difficult?

- Have you ever wished you could play a game without keeping score?

- Can you have a good game (play well) and still lose?

- Can you have fun even when you lose?

- What's an example of a game you played that was a lot of fun even though you lost?

Fallen Heroes / Drugs

These so-called heroes are constantly providing parents and coaches with opportunities to talk to their athletes about what *not* to do. Every time you turn around, there's another athlete in the headlines with allegations of steroid use, recreational drug use, drunk driving, domestic violence, rape, and even murder. It would be really easy to start a list of professional athletes who have destroyed their careers.

Don't ignore this teaching opportunity. When someone your child admires does something stupid, it's a good opportunity to talk about what you admire in other people. What makes someone a good role model? What about this "hero" impresses your child? Encourage them to find additional role models closer to home, people they really know.

A growing problem in sports is the prevalence of performance-enhancing drugs, and these drugs represent the ultimate loss of perspective in sports. Users are taking enormous health risks for performance benefits gained unfairly. Some will attempt to excuse the use with the "everyone's doing it" rationale, that they have to use drugs in order to level the playing field. Be clear that using drugs is against the rules. When you play sports, you're accepting the rules of the game. Cheating with drugs is no different than cutting a race course.

Problems that surface at the professional level work their way down. With millions of dollars at stake, it shouldn't surprise anyone that drug use is rampant. When the pros get away with using drugs, it trickles down to the college and high school levels. The surprising thing is this: Money and fame are not the only motives for drug users. Drug use in amateur competitions is undocumented because, for the most part, no testing programs are in place. There are even people who take drugs to have the ego trip of being the strongest guy in their local gym or the winner of a local race.

ShadowBuster:

Talk to your child early and often about the dangers of drugs. Don't assume it won't happen to them or those around them. If you talk about drugs from an athletic perspective early on, it will make it easier to talk to them about other types of drugs that make their appearance in junior high and high school. Be clear that no achievement is worth sacrificing long-term health or personal integrity.

ShadowBuster Questions

- Why do people cheat?

- What fulfillment could possibly be gained by cheating one's way to victory?

- Would you rather get second on your own or first with "help"?

- Would you rather get a "B" that you legitimately earned or cheat your way to an "A" grade?

- Is it OK to cheat if "everyone is doing it?" Why or why not?

Destructive Attitudes

Some kids don't enjoy sports because they haven't found one they're good at, and every team has members who like nothing better than to tear someone else down. When the target is the less-talented child on the team, this certainly compounds the problem of a bad attitude. Have your child try different sports until they discover one they enjoy. Once your child finds a sport they enjoy, be prepared to stick with it long enough for them to improve. If they're constantly jumping from one sport to another and are behind their peers in size and coordination, they may come away with the impression that they "aren't good at anything."

It's important for them to want success. If they don't care about sports enough to go to practice and want to improve, then they simply aren't going to get any better. If they truly don't care about performance, find an activity that they can do in order to meet the minimum requirement; then it won't matter if they're "good" at it or not. If the focus is strictly on health and not on the sport, it really doesn't matter what they're doing or how well they're doing it. At least they're out from in front of the TV and are active enough to stay healthy. As someone somewhere once said: "If you can't learn to do something well, learn to enjoy doing it poorly!"

ShadowBuster:

Make it clear that your child is expected to play a sport whether they're "good" at sports or not. If they aren't "good" at reading, what do you do? You get them help so they can survive in the classroom and the real world. You don't expect them to love reading and curl up with a good book for hours on end; they just have to do it well enough to keep up at school and prepare for the future. They have to do enough physical activity, whether they like it or not, to keep them fit and healthy.

ShadowBuster Questions:

- What are three things you're good at?

- Who's the best athlete your age that you know?

- How do you know if you're good at something?

- What are some specific things you can do to improve at something you don't think you're good at?

- What are some specific things you can do to improve at something you know you're already good at?

Division / Cliques / Infighting

Many of us have had the experience of being part of a great team. Some of those teams were sports related, some of them weren't. It's a lot of fun to be surrounded by a great group of people all avidly pursuing the same goal. However, we've also all been on "teams" where this wasn't the case. Maybe it was a study group where some of the members refused to pull their weight or a team at work that degenerated into uncooperative factions. Maybe it was a sports team that fell apart and lost sight of their goals.

Many times, petty disagreements and miscommunication take on a life of their own; they spiral out of control and destroy the chances of a successful season. This disunity can take many different forms. It can be two players feuding, causing the rest of the team to take sides. It can also be the team uniting against the coach and self-destructing in the process.

During my senior year of high school, I ran cross-country. It was a difficult semester because I was participating in both swimming and cross-country and competing, on average, four days a week. I was fortunate enough to have coaches who allowed me to split my time between the two sports. It was an incredible blessing for me that the school got a new cross-country coach that season, Don Giardina. Unfortunately, the rest of the team didn't see it that way.

This team was the most dedicated group I had ever been involved with. While swimmers I had trained with often looked for any excuse to skip a practice, the cross-country team would be meeting on their own without a coach every day in the summer at 6:00 in the morning to run up to an hour and a half. Though it was a great group of guys who were very supportive of the team and each other, they just didn't believe in the new coach. They had been used to doing things a certain way with the old coach and they didn't want to change. Though we had a great season, the team collapsed at State, placing fourth when we should have won. At the end of the season, during the awards party, the captains broke down in tears with the realization that if they had believed in Don's program, we would have been celebrating a state championship. Don coached at the high school for three more years and even though that first year had the most talent, he won state championships two of the next three years with lesser talent that bonded together to create a better team.

ShadowBuster:

First, sit down with your child and write a list of what makes a good team. Talk to your child about what sports teams they admire. Ask them why these teams are great teams. Use the many examples of high-profile clubhouse feuds in the professional ranks to show how one person or a number of people can damage the whole of a team. What does it take to move beyond a collection of great players and make a great team? Team building is a skill that certainly has the potential to carry over to "real life." Corporate America is a study of how teams work in business. It takes a great team to make a great company. If everyone on the team is constantly fighting amongst themselves, they're not going to be successful. If people are more concerned about making themselves look good, about trying to make themselves the star, the performance of the team is going to suffer.

Second, observe how your child acts toward the coach and the team during practices and games. Are they part of the problem or part of the solution? Do they really understand what it means to be part of the team? Do they know what it means to put the needs of the team ahead of the needs of an individual? Do they not just accept, but understand why they might not be able to play their favorite position because the team needs them to play somewhere else?

Third, be ready to ask for help. Don't let a situation get to the point where it's beyond repair. Talk to the coach as soon as you see a problem or potential problem. Work with the coach, your child, and the other parents on the team. Everyone on the team has the same goal (or should have the same goal), and that's where leadership comes in.

ShadowBuster Questions:
- What makes a good team? What makes a great team?

- Describe one game that your team played that was an example of a perfect team performance.

- If you could change one thing about your team, what would it be?

- What can you do at your next practice or game that would make the team better?

Plateau / Declining Performance

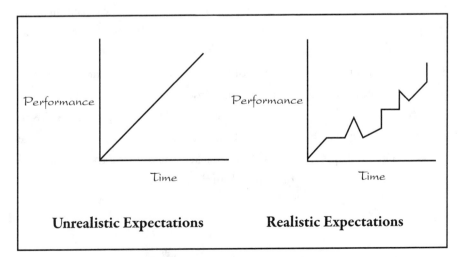

Unrealistic Expectations   **Realistic Expectations**

Improvement in sports is a lot like the stock market. Overall, if an athlete stays in a sport, they're going to continue to improve in the long term barring any major changes in body type. Certain types of athletes have their window of opportunity earlier than others; you may see gymnasts, skaters, runners, or swimmers (particularly females) who will have a better performance in their sport before they mature into their adult body. For most other athletes, the improvement is going to come in the long run. If you pick any stock right now and invest some money in it, forty years from now it will likely be worth a lot more as long as the company is still around. Progress is not a linear function.

The problem enters into the equation when you use recent performance to predict short-term results. In the tech stock run-up of the late nineties, people assumed that the value of these stocks would continue to rise at their current rate forever, an observation that in hindsight we know couldn't have possibly been maintained. In sports that are quantified by times, such as swimming or running, you can't use the results of one good meet to predict that if your child goes a second faster every month, in two years they'll make the Olympics. That's just not the way it works.

Athletes in all sports tend to plateau, and then make a giant leap forward. In professional sports, it's often called the "sophomore slump." Many athletes will have a great rookie season, and then follow it up with a terrible second year. Your child needs to understand there are peaks and valleys. It's just not possible to sustain a constant rate of improvement, especially with the developmental changes that occur as a child grows. Depending on their rate of growth, it's as if they're competing in a different body every year or every couple months. It's difficult to maintain balance and coordination in a body that's constantly changing. Once they're done growing, they lose those performance boosts that come from a bigger body and must work even harder to make smaller gains in performance. This is where the curse of early success comes back into play. The better you get at a sport, the harder and harder it is to make the incremental improvements. Progress is not a linear function.

ShadowBuster:

Teach your child to take the peaks and valleys in stride. Although they need to celebrate their successes, they also need to learn something from defeats and beware of dwelling too much on the past. Help them focus on the present and what they can do now to put themselves in a position to achieve their goals.

Sometimes goals change slightly, and other times they change radically. In 2005, Jim MacLaren won a share of the Arthur Ashe Courage Award at the ESPY sports awards. He was a scholar at Yale and a football star when he was hit by a bus at the age of twenty-two, nearly died and lost his left leg below the knee. He started swimming, then picked up cycling and running with the aid of a prosthetic and became one of the pre-eminent amputee athletes in the world. He regularly finished in the top 20 percent and he set amputee records in the marathon as well as the Ironman Triathlon. When he was thirty, he was struck by a van while cycling in a triathlon and became a quadriplegic. After cheating death the second time, he faced the prospect of life in a wheelchair without any sensation below the neck. Here's an example of circumstances that can cause goals to change drastically. Rather than give up on life completely, Jim formed the Choose Living Foundation and continues to work on his rehabilitation. He has regained sensation all over his body and regained the use of his arms. Rather than drown himself in the well of self-pity, he has gone on to make a difference for untold thousands of people and has discovered the joy of helping other people reach their goals.

Though this is an extreme example, it shows how one man changed his goals and stayed involved in a sport. External circumstances prevented him from achieving his original goals on two separate tragic occasions. Rather than abandon sports completely, he changed his goal to fit the new reality and became far more successful than he otherwise could have been.

ShadowBuster Questions:

- Are you happy with your performance this season?

- What can you do better to improve for next season?

- What is your goal in your sport?

- If you don't achieve your goal, then what?

Unhealthy Obsession

When does a healthy activity morph into an unhealthy obsession? Though sports can help to focus your child and provide incentive to manage their time well, it can also consume their life. In my experience, the more I have to do, the more I get done. Even during times of heavy training, I'm rarely overwhelmed to the point where everything suffers. I find that when I'm training, I'm amazed at how productive I am on a given day. Conversely, during the brief off season, I'm surprised at how little I'm able to get done. It seems that the more time I have, the more time I waste. I think devoting so much time to sports growing up actually allowed me to get a lot more out of my childhood.

There comes a point where you must determine what the appropriate level of involvement is for your child. Obsession is OK, unhealthy obsession is not. You'll find that most great athletes have to be obsessed with their sport, just as many successful businessmen are obsessed with work. In order to rise to the top of a very competitive field, you have to be willing to do things, make commitments and sacrifices that other people aren't willing to do. The key is to keep referring to your child's goals. To what end? Help your child understand what's right for them. The way you approach sports will be vastly different if the goal is to play on a Division I college team as opposed to participating to enjoy being with friends and stay fit.

ShadowBuster:

Even when a goal becomes an obsession, it's important to keep perspective. I've mentioned two goals that became obsessions for me, lasting six years each: competing in the Ironman Triathlon in 1998 and winning the Rhodes Scholarship in 2002. I was able to deal very well with the Rhodes failure because the Ironman goal had allowed me to see that the eventual results didn't tell the whole tale about the worth of the goal and the investment of time when single-mindedly pursuing a dream. Pursuing a goal isn't about what you will do or what you will get, but who you will become in the process. Teach your child not to judge success or failure based on the achievement of their ultimate goal.

ShadowBuster Questions:

- What are you *not* doing now that you wish you had time to do?

- If you had to give up one activity you're doing now, what would it be?

- What's your favorite time of the week?

- If you could accomplish anything, what would it be?

- If you failed to do that (above), what's something that you might learn while pursuing your goal that would make you a better person?

Chapter Summary

By shining light into the shadows of sports, you can be fully aware of the destructive side and do your best to keep the experience positive for your child. Kids quit sports for reasons that go beyond "it's too hard" or "it's not fun." These shadows are what make it "not fun" or "too hard." In order to conquer the shadows, recognize and deal with the negative aspects of sports. Work together with your child, the coach, and the team in answering the ShadowBuster Questions to turn the negatives into positives.

CHAPTER TEN

COMMON SENSE NUTRITION

▲

Joe's Rule #10: "Properly fuel the fire."

I've spent a lifetime in sports and I believe that nutrition is the most overlooked component of a successful athletic program. In the previous nine chapters, we've looked at all the benefits of sports participation; without proper nutrition, some of those benefits will be completely negated. It's important enough to devote an entire chapter to the topic. I am not a nutritionist. I don't have an advanced degree in nutrition and I don't, personally, have a whole lot of scientific evidence to back up this chapter. That's why it's called common sense nutrition. There are many books about nutrition written by people who have lots of letters after their name, and there are several good books that deal specifically with the topic of nutrition for young athletes. However, a book about getting the most out of sports would be incomplete without this chapter. Sports activity without proper nutrition is like putting the lowest grade of gasoline in a car you're racing. You can build up that body of a car to be a real beauty, but when it comes time for the engine to roar to life, you're not going to get the performance you deserve without the right fuel.

A Balanced Diet

The most important thing about nutrition is to eat a balanced diet. All three of the macronutrients—carbohydrates, proteins, and fats—are good for you. That's why they're called nutrients. You just have to be smart about what your child is eating. Calories are the small energy units the body uses all through the day, and they're in every type of food. If you don't use this energy contained in the food, it's stored by the body for later use; in other words, it ends up stored as fat, or in athletes as glycogen.

Carbohydrates

Carbohydrates are your body's source of glucose. Glucose is a simple carbohydrate that is stored in your muscles as glycogen. Glucose is easily obtained by your body and is easily stored, so it is used to fuel most of your body's cells. There are complex carbohydrates, foods with a low glycemic index that are good for you. Complex carbohydrates are found in whole grains, cereals, oat bran, vegetables, rice, and pasta. Simple carbohydrates are the simple sugars that you want to eat in moderation. They are best used for recovery; after a workout, simple carbohydrates will help to replenish glycogen stores. Simple carbohydrates are found in white flour, white pasta, baked goods, and fruit juice. If your child isn't eating enough carbohydrates, the body will start to break down muscle tissue for glucose since glucose can be made from protein.

Proteins

Proteins affect the repairing, replacing, and growing of tissue. With a young, growing athlete, the intake of protein is especially important because they need that protein to fuel growth. Protein intake must exceed output for the body to have the fuel to add muscle. If your protein output is greater than the intake, it puts your body in a catabolic state. A catabolic state is where body compounds are broken down to be used for energy. You cannot grow if your body is constantly in a catabolic state. This is why eating immediately after a workout, including some protein, is so important. If your body is in a catabolic state instead of an anabolic state, you cannot get the most benefit from your training. Healthy foods high in protein include eggs, soy products, tofu, legumes, fish, peanut butter, and lean meats.

Fats

Body fat stores are the main source of energy when athletes are working in an aerobic capacity—that is, working at a low intensity for a prolonged period of time. This does NOT mean that your child should eat foods high in fat to give them energy during periods of aerobic exercise. During aerobic exercise, the human body will burn the fat stores it already has. Body fat stores and glucose from dietary carbohydrates and/or muscle glycogen are utilized for energy production.

Saturated fat should be limited in your child's diet because the body makes cholesterol from saturated fat and is more likely to store saturated fat as body fat. Unsaturated fat is better because it's easy for the body to break down and use with carbohydrates and proteins to function optimally. Good sources of unsaturated fat are liquid vegetable oils and fish. If you eat too much of anything, it's stored as fat.

Individualized Nutrition

The nutrition needs of a young athlete can be very specific. Rather than just rely on a one-size-fits-all mantra that you might hear from another person or read in a magazine, it's worth setting up an appointment with a dietitian to find out your child's specific nutrition needs and how best to meet those needs.

Nutrition is, perhaps, the most frustrating part of my training. In swimming, cycling, and running, there are generally accepted guidelines for training that most everyone agrees lead to peak performance. Nutrition is a different story. For the last twelve years, I've seen all kinds of conflicting information out there. At one point, I heard that athletes should eat a lot of carbs and engage in "carbo-loading" before an event. Then I heard that it should be the 40/30/30 or "zone diet" and that "carbo-loading" is detrimental. Shortly after, I heard that a vegetarian diet is the only healthy way to go, then that the high-fat "Atkins" diet or one that is high in protein is the answer. I got to the point where I finally gave up and established my own guidelines of what has worked for me

Sports activity without proper nutrition is like putting the lowest grade of gasoline in a car you're building for peak performance.

in the past and some general ideas of what makes for healthy eating and peak performance.

The Ironman Triathlon has been called an "eating contest." Because so many of the top athletes in the world all have similar genetic talent and similar training background, the winner is usually the person who can get the most out of his body on the day of the competition. On any given day, there are about a dozen men in the professional field that, given their perfect race, could walk away the winner. In a race that lasts over eight hours in extremely hot, humid, and windy conditions, properly fueling the fire makes all the difference. Now most of us don't go around racing 140.6 miles on a given day, but your child's day (whatever it is they're doing) lasts even longer than those eight hours. In order to be at their peak during the day, they must have the proper fuel.

Eating for Success

Eating for success involves two facets: eating for performance and general, everyday healthy eating. There's an obvious equation to maintain a given weight. Calories in must equal calories out. If your child is regularly consuming more calories than they are burning, then they're going to put on weight. Beyond the actual number of calories, it's important that they be from the right types of food.

General, Everyday Healthy Eating

When I'm racing in a triathlon, the goal is to keep the glucose in my blood at a constant level. I eat when I'm not hungry and I drink when I'm not thirsty, because the water you drink today keeps you hydrated for tomorrow. If I wait until I start to feel starved and dehydrated, it's too late to catch up on my nutrition. I plan my daily nutrition the same way. Every time glucose levels spike from eating a lot of sugar, there is going to be a valley where the level bottoms out. If your child is constantly alternating between a peak and a valley, they're not going to be having a very good day.

The day should start with a good breakfast. Rushing out the door and downing some Pop Tarts on the way isn't a very good start. Get your child up ten minutes earlier if that's what it takes. Start with some whole grains, protein, fruit, and water. The first thing I do when I get up every morning is drink a glass of water. You wake up every morning dehydrated since you haven't had anything to drink in the last six to nine hours. Make proper nutrition a priority in the morning. For kids, the effect is even greater. Because they sleep longer, by the time they get up in the morning, they haven't eaten in perhaps twelve to fourteen hours. Their bodies are in a state of starvation and dehydration; they need to counter that with a good nutritional start to the day.

It seems that schools are having lunch earlier and earlier. It's not uncommon to have a lunch period at 10:30 in the morning. After a healthy lunch, make sure there's a good snack waiting for them after school. If they have practice after school, it's vital that there's something between their early school lunch and practice. When kids tell me that they're tired, the first thing I ask is what they had for lunch and how long ago they last ate. My follow-up question is what they've been drinking since lunch. It's not uncommon for them to feel tired and sick because it's 5:30 and the last thing they ate was pizza at lunch (over five hours ago). The only thing they've had to drink is soda. They're wondering why they don't feel well, and I'm wondering how they can still function given the circumstances. Be sure to send your child to school with a healthy lunch (for example, a sandwich with lean turkey, lettuce, and tomato on whole wheat or grain bread).

The first thirty minutes after practice is the most important time to be eating and drinking. If your child isn't going to have dinner for an hour or more after a practice, it would be helpful to have something small (like a banana or granola bar) right after practice. The body is depleted after working out and will soak up anything that's provided. After a workout is the ideal time to consume a sports drink to replenish the electrolytes from sweat losses.

The most overlooked part of a healthy diet is what your kids are drinking.

Drinks like fruit juice, punches, and soda are loaded with calories. They're liquid candy bars. A can of soda has the equivalent of ten teaspoons of sugar. Try an experiment: Take a twelve-ounce glass of water and then dump ten teaspoons of sugar into it. Because it's dissolved in water, the sugar high takes effect much more quickly than if it were in a food. Look at the nutrition information of the beverages that your family drinks and see if it's conducive to an overall healthy lifestyle. If a drink screams that it's "made with real fruit juice" and you see that it has 10 percent juice, then in that twelve-ounce can is approximately 1.2 ounces of juice. That's less than a shot of juice mixed into ten ounces of sugar water, not exactly a healthy alternative to soda.

Eating and drinking right isn't always the easy thing to do. It can be difficult, time consuming, and expensive. But it's important. If you think of all the money you spend on school and sports-related activities, it's well worth the investment to make sure your children are properly fueled for their activities.

Eating for Performance

The first rule of thumb is don't try anything new right before a competition. A lot of people ask me what I eat the night before a triathlon and the morning of a triathlon. The night before, I have salad and spaghetti (or similar pasta), and in the morning I have a bagel and a banana. I try to eat a big meal the night before so that I'm not very hungry in the morning. This is what I've found works well for me. I don't pretend that it will work for everyone.

I also make sure I'm well-hydrated the night before. "Hyper-hydrating" several days out is generally a waste of time because your body will flush out the excess water well in advance of the race. It's important to hydrate with a sports drink rather than exclusively with water. By over-hydrating with water, you risk flushing out the salts and electrolytes that your body needs to perform at your best.

As usual, the answer is moderation. There is no "magic bullet" food that works for everyone before a race. It's important to find what works for your child, and once you find a good mix of foods, then stick with it. Before a game or between games, you want to avoid foods that are high in sugar, caffeine, protein, or fat. It is best to consume mainly carbohydrates with small amounts of protein.

It's especially important to eat well in the period of time leading up to a major competition. The few days before and the night before are vital because that's going to be the food that fuels your child during the competition. In my swimming career, I've heard two opposite extremes from coaches. One stressed staying away from sugar at all costs going into a meet, and another said, "Eat what makes you happy because happy swimmers swim fast." The right answer lies somewhere between those two views. It's important to eat right all the time and even more important to be smart about nutrition in the days leading up to a big event.

When your child is going to a meet that lasts for several hours or a tournament that features several games played over the course of the day, make sure you plan their eating ahead of time. Know what food is available in and around the venue. Typically, the food served at concession stands is horrible for you. If you can't find a restaurant for a good lunch between games, make sure you bring your own food.

Nutrition is important, but it's not magic. I can remember times when I would come back in the evening for the final session of a swim meet and a teammate was telling me that he had two burgers, fries, and a milkshake for lunch. Meanwhile, I had plain pasta and bread, and he'd still smoke me in the pool. Though nutrition may not make the difference in outperforming someone else, it will allow your child to perform at their personal best, which is the ultimate goal.

Eating Right at School

When I was in college, I worked as a lunchroom monitor in a junior high school. It was so much more fun than it sounds! I thought of it a lot like lifeguarding. I'm convinced I learned as much there as I did in my psychology classes. One of the things I noticed was how many of the kids had a bag of Doritos and a can of Mountain Dew from the vending machines for lunch. This wasn't a one-time "I forgot my lunch" occurrence. This was an everyday pattern.

I had to wonder what these kids were eating during the rest of the day. If they had a bowl of Froot Loops for breakfast, chips and soda for lunch, and a similar type of snack food after school, they'd put themselves so far behind that no matter what dinner was, the day was an unmitigated disaster from a nutrition standpoint. People wonder why their kids can't pay attention in school, and I'm wondering how they can even sit still after seeing what they eat for lunch. The only thing that shocked me more than seeing "lunch" was seeing the nurse's office and how many of the kids were on mood-altering drugs. Now, I'm not a doctor (at least not yet), but maybe there's a simpler answer than what the pharmaceutical companies are offering. Maybe if you eliminated the constant blood-sugar spikes and caffeine-induced highs, some of the behavioral problems could be explained.

Eating right starts at home. As a child gets older and their leash gets longer, they have to take on more responsibility for their nutrition. But in the meantime, model and teach healthy eating habits for your children at home. The more they understand why certain food is good for them and how particular foods affect them, the more likely they are to make better choices for themselves when given the chance.

Kids And Sports Drinks

One problem with many sports drinks is that they have a lot of sugar in them. For many young athletes, the events they participate in aren't long enough for them to really need the extra salts and electrolytes that a sports drink provides. There's also some evidence that sports drinks can contribute to kidney stones for children who are prone to that. Most commercial sports drinks are formulated for a person who weighs 150 pounds. Giving the same drink to a child who weighs half of that probably is not their best choice for hydration. Until the introduction of a "kids formula" sports drink, it's best to dilute a sports drink so they're still getting some of the salts and electrolytes, but not too much of it at once.

If the period of exercise is prolonged or if conditions lend themselves to a lot of sweating, then a diluted sports drink is probably the best idea. Sports drinks taste better so kids will drink more than if water is the only drink available. The importance of hydration cannot be overrated. In all sports, kids should bring their own water bottle to practice regardless of the sport and weather conditions. Though hot weather presents the most danger of dehydration, the effects of training in cool weather can be insidious because you don't feel as thirsty even though the water loss due to exercise continues. If kids are feeling excessively tired during practice, have a headache, or are suffering muscle cramps, dehydration could be contributing to these conditions.

Junk Food / Desserts

The key is to do everything in moderation. When I'm in heavy training, there aren't any foods I enjoy that I avoid completely. When I'm tapering, preparing for a major competition, I make sure that I taper my eating as well. Eating is a habit. I have to consciously cut down on the amount of calories I take in when I'm not in heavy training. While I might have no problem having dessert (or even two desserts) as I'm struggling to keep the weight on while training six hours a day, I'll skip dessert when I'm on taper and preparing to peak for a major event.

Eating junk food is a lot like watching TV. In limited amounts, it's not going to cause a problem. When it becomes part of the everyday habit, then you have something to worry about. Besides television and junk food contributing to inactivity and poor eating habits, they feed on each other. Watch the commercials that come on during programming aimed at children and prepare to be amazed at the number of advertisements for junk food. Sitting on the couch, eating junk food while watching TV is the double whammy. If that's a common occurrence in your household, something has to change!

What Happens When My Kid Gains Weight?

A small weight gain isn't cause for concern because it will often be followed by a growth spurt that will cause them to lose the fat. Even if their numerical weight doesn't decline, their increased size will lower the body mass index.

If it's more than a small weight gain, realize this: They didn't gain the weight overnight and they won't lose it overnight. There are a number of kids who may be spending a lot of time being active, but are still carrying around a lot more weight than they should. In that case, diet and nutrition have to take on primary importance. You don't want to necessarily restrict the amount of food that a child eats, but rather the types of food. The most important thing for weight loss is for kids to want to lose the weight. It's going to be very difficult to force a diet on them because you can't watch them every hour of every day. They have to see for themselves how much more fun it is to have a body that feels good and can allow them to experience life. Nobody wants to be fat. The desire to maintain a healthy weight must outweigh the desire to eat certain foods.

Power Foods / Vitamins / Supplements

There's a huge market now for energy bars. Energy bars can be a great snack for after school and before sports. They're easy enough to transport and are balanced with a good amount of pre-training nutrition. They come in a variety of brands and flavors, and when coupled with a piece of fruit and a bottle of water, they can provide the calories needed to make it through a practice. Take the time to read labels and understand what is in the food you're putting into your body.

Don't look to foods, however, as a performance enhancer. While it's common to use a drug like caffeine to "get up" for a game, it's not a good idea for the long term. Like any drug, it takes more and more to get the same results, and if it's part of the routine, it can become a mental addiction more than a physical one.

A daily vitamin may be a good way to "fill in the gaps" of a daily diet. It's important to look for the "USP" label on vitamins. This indicates that the brand in question meets the standards of the U.S. Pharmacopeia testing organization. Vitamins are not "food substitutes" and should not be considered the magic bullet to balance out otherwise unhealthy food choices. Best plan: check with your pediatrician.

Kids Need to be Involved in Their Nutrition

Eating habits will make the difference between a healthy weight and obesity.

The most important part of any nutrition program is to get your child to buy into it. There has to be a reason, a motivation for doing it. You can stand there all day telling them that they should eat a food they hate because "it's good for you" or not eat a food they like because "it's bad for you," but until they believe it for themselves, it's not going to be as effective. If you pay attention, it's pretty apparent how nutrition correlates with mood. When someone's hungry or thirsty, they're usually irritable. Point out to your child how different foods affect their moods, behavior, ability to sleep, and ability to concentrate. If your child is excited about sports and is earnestly trying to improve their skills, make sure they understand how nutrition plays a role in how they perform.

Chapter Summary

Proper nutrition and eating right isn't about looking a certain way or fitting into a certain size of clothes, it's about health and building the foundation for a healthy lifestyle. In the long run, eating habits will make the difference between a healthy weight and obesity. The human body wasn't built to handle the amounts of weight people are packing on today. Hips, knees, and ankles weren't designed to handle the constant stress of an extra fifty or a hundred pounds.

Remember to plan ahead. Your child can eat right and eat well if you think ahead and work at it. Most of the "easy" foods to find and eat are not what you want them to be eating for optimal performance. Model healthy eating by bringing the right kinds of food into your house. They can't eat it if you don't have it.

Costs associated with preventative health care are always a good investment. Participating in sports is not cheap, and a health club membership isn't cheap. Buying healthy foods and taking the time to prepare them have costs as well. However, when you take into account the costs associated with the alternative (medical expenses, illness, obesity, and a general sense of malaise), the costs of a healthy lifestyle pale in comparison.

CALL TO ACTION

Now that you're aware of how important it is for your child to play sports and have a positive experience doing so, it's time to **do something** about it. The following questions are meant to reinforce the critical role you play as a parent. They'll assist you in getting to know your child's goals, hopes, and dreams so you can help them create a positive vision for the future. Remember, it's not about what your child will do or what your child will have. It's about who they will become. In the process of answering the following questions, you'll make yourself a better person. Go ahead and be your child's greatest hero.

1. **What's my child's genius?**
   My child is particularly talented at...

   _____

   _____

   _____

   _____

   _____

   _____

   _____

My child most enjoys...

_____

_____

_____

_____

_____

_____

Participation in sports will help unlock my child's genius because...

_____

_____

_____

_____

_____

_____

2. **How can sports benefit my child?**

On the spectrum of *Laid-Back to Intense*, "laid-back" being a "1" and "intense" being a "10," my child is about a _____.

Participation in sports will help my child...

On the spectrum of *Nervous to Confident*, "nervous" being a "1" and "confident" being a "10," my child is about a _____.

Participation in sports will help my child...

On the spectrum of *Thinker to Doer*, "thinker" being a "1" and "doer" being a "10," my child is about a _____.

Participation in sports will help my child...

Rate the following benefits in order, from what matters most to you (1) to what matters least (10). Then have your child rate the benefits based on what matters most to them.

_____ Emotional and Mental Well-Being

_____ Lessons from Your Own Regrets

_____ Keeping Them Busy

_____ Fitness for Life

_____ Fun and Friends

_____ Being Part of a Team

_____ Independence

_____ Competition

_____ Discipline and Self-Confidence

_____ Elite/Collegiate/Professional Athletic Goals

My goal for my child's participation in sports:

_____

_____

_____

_____

_____

I will know this goal is being met because I can measure it by...

_____

_____

_____

_____

_____

_____

The following is my child's goal:

_____

_____

_____

_____

_____

_____

My child will know this goal is being met because it can be measured by...

_____

_____

_____

_____

_____

3. **What sport, level, and program is right for my child?**
    What sport is my child interested in?

_____

_____

_____

_____

_____

_____

What sport am I interested in for my child?

_____

_____

_____

_____

_____

Which of the following stages is my child in?

_____

_____

_____

_____

_____

Put a check next to the appropriate answer.

_____ Stage 1: Moving and Learning (Age 6 & Under)

_____ Stage 2: The Big World (Age 7-9)

_____ Stage 3: Decision Time (Age 10-12)

_____ Stage 4: Impending Specialization (Age 12-15)

_____ Stage 5: Specialization (Age 14 & Up)

What type of program would fit my child right now?

Put a check next to the appropriate answer.

_____ Recreational Sports

_____ Competitive Sports

_____ School Sports

When I'm considering a program for my child, I'm looking for the following when it comes to:

The coach...

The atmosphere...

Skill development...

Philosophy and vision...

4. **What type of coach and team would be best for my child?**
    Put a check next to the appropriate answer.

_____ My goal is: Participation for Health
    So, this is what I'm looking for in a coach and team...

_____ My goal is: Participation for Fitness
    So, this is what I'm looking for in a coach and team...

_____ My goal is: Participation for Performance
    So, this is what I'm looking for in a coach and team...

Rate yourself on a scale of 1-10 (1 being never, 10 being always).

_____ I avoid treating my child like a professional athlete.

_____ I'm patient and positive.

_____ I recognize that "The Coach is the Coach."

_____ I prepare my child for success off the field.

_____ I help my child understand that it won't always be fun.

_____ I help my child understand that it's OK to try things they aren't comfortable with.

_____ I help my child understand that it's OK to feel discouraged and defeated.

_____ Even if I'm not sure what to do, at least I'm doing something.

_____ I don't allow my child to quit a sport without having an answer to "quit to do what?"

Considering the above ratings I gave myself, my goal is:

_____

_____

_____

_____

_____

_____

I will know whether or not I'm meeting my goal because I can measure it by...

_____

_____

_____

_____

_____

5. **What motivates my child?**
   My child is motivated by the following.
   Put a check next to the appropriate answer(s).

   _____Friendship

   _____Awards

   _____Personal Improvement

   _____Praise

   _____Competition

   _____Rewards

My child has the following type of motivation personality.
Put a check next to the appropriate answer.

_____ The Flameout
Now that I realize this, I can help my child by...

_____ The Slow to Warm Up
Now that I realize this, I can help my child by...

_____ The Optimally Motivated
Now that I realize this, I can help my child by...

_____ The Under-Motivated
Now that I realize this, I can help my child by...

_____ The Unmotivated that I realize this, I can help my child by...
Now do I "push" or "pull" my child? How do I know?

6. Is my child maintaining balance?

Put a check next to the appropriate answer.

_____ My child seems to be balancing sports, school, and their other activities/responsibilities.

This is how I know...

This is how I can help them maintain the balance...

_____ My child seems to be having trouble balancing sports, school, and their other activities/responsibilities.

This is how I know...

_____

_____

_____

_____

This is how I can help them regain balance...

_____

_____

_____

_____

_____

_____

7. Is my child exposed to healthy competition?

What's my attitude toward competition?

_____

_____

_____

_____

_____

Is my focus on the *foundation* for results (talent, technique, and conditioning) or solely on the results?

_____

_____

_____

_____

_____

_____

When I focus on results, are they results my child has control over?

_____

_____

_____

_____

_____

_____

Does my child understand the connection between effort and results? How do I know?

_____

_____

_____

_____

_____

_____

Does my child have opportunities to experience winning?

_____

_____

_____

_____

_____

Does my child have opportunities to lose and learn from it?

_____

_____

_____

_____

_____

8. **Am I making sure my child's participation in sports is shaping their character in a positive way?**

    Does my child display good SPORTSMANSHIP?

    Yes _____ No _____ Sometimes _____

    How can I accentuate this positive?

    Does my child get to CELEBRATE SUCCESSES?
    Yes _____ No _____ Sometimes _____

    How can I accentuate this positive?

    Does my child have ROLE MODELS AND HEROES?

    Yes _____ No _____

    How can I accentuate this positive?

    Do sports play in my child's SELF-PERCEPTION?

    Yes _____ No _____

    How can I accentuate this positive?

    Does my child understand what it means to be part of a TEAM?

    Yes _____ No _____

How can I accentuate this positive?

Is my child having FUN?

    Yes _____ No _____

How can I accentuate this positive?

_____

_____

_____

_____

_____

_____

Is my child experiencing SKILL DEVELOPMENT AND IMPROVEMENT?

    Yes _____ No _____

How can I accentuate this positive?

Does my child have A HEALTHY LIFESTYLE?

    Yes _____ No _____

How can I accentuate this positive?

_____

_____

_____

_____

_____

9. **Am I helping minimize the negatives for my child?**
    Do I talk with my child about POOR SPORTSMANSHIP and turn those opportunities into teachable moments?

    Yes _____ No _____ Sometimes _____

    Do I talk with my child about OVER-EMPHASIS ON RESULTS ("WIN AT ALL COSTS") and turn those opportunities into teachable moments?

    Yes _____ No _____ Sometimes _____

    Do I talk with my child about FALLEN HEROES / DRUGS and turn those opportunities into teachable moments?

    Yes _____ No _____ Sometimes _____

    Do I talk with my child about DESTRUCTIVE ATTITUDES and turn those opportunities into teachable moments?

    Yes _____ No _____ Sometimes _____

    Do I talk with my child about DIVISION / CLIQUES / INFIGHTING and turn those opportunities into teachable moments?

    Yes _____ No _____ Sometimes _____

    Do I talk with my child about PLATEAU / DECLINING PERFORMANCE and turn those opportunities into teachable moments?

    Yes _____ No _____ Sometimes _____

    Do I talk with my child about UNHEALTHY OBSESSION and turn those opportunities into teachable moments?

    Yes _____ No _____ Sometimes _____

My goal to help minimize the negative:

_____

_____

_____

_____

_____

_____

I will know I'm meeting this goal because I can measure it by:

_____

_____

_____

_____

_____

_____

10. **Am I teaching my child common sense nutrition and properly fueling the fire?**

What does my child eat for breakfast?

_____

_____

_____

_____

_____

What does my child eat for lunch?

_____

_____

_____

_____

_____

What does my child eat for dinner?

_____

_____

_____

_____

_____

Do I model healthy eating?

_____

_____

_____

_____

_____

_____

Does my child eat a healthy snack before and after practice or a game?

_____

_____

_____

_____

Does my child understand the impact healthy eating has on mood, energy, and performance?

_____

_____

_____

_____

My goal for creating better eating habits for my child:

_____

_____

_____

_____

I will know I'm meeting this goal because I can measure it by...

_____

_____

_____

_____

Afterword

As this book goes to print—nearly one year to the day that Braxton set a new world record at Alcatraz—and I look back on the past twelve months, I cannot believe the strides we've made.

Braxton has inspired over fifty of his teammates to make a 2007 Alcatraz swim to focus national and international attention on childhood drowning prevention. Team Alcatraz is training now—an incredible group of boys and girls with both personal and team goals... motivated by an unassuming eight-year-old. Coaching this team has been a coach's dream.

Swim Neptune, a competitive year-round USA Swimming program, has grown to include five locations across the Phoenix metro area and continues to nurture young swimmers in their competitive goals. The Inaugural Mayoral Race, slated for summer 2007 in Phoenix, will provide yet another springboard to furthering the cause of water safety and training.

People from across the country who watch these young swimmers grow and excel ask me how they can "bring Swim Neptune to their communities"... and a plan for that is taking shape.

Most important of all, perhaps, has been the evolution of F.A.S.T.—The Foundation for Aquatic Safety and Training. A non-profit organization, based in Phoenix, F.A.S.T. was inspired by Braxton's commitment and tenacity and his goal of preventing childhood drownings.

It's been said that a worthy goal is to "serve the many." That has been my goal in writing *Joe's Rules*. This book, and all the *Joe's Rules* books to follow, will carry important messages farther and faster than I, or any one person, can ever hope to.

To the millions of young people the world over whose lives can be enriched through sports, I challenge you. To parents—and friends and grandparents and mentors and family members and teachers—who look to this book for guidance and support in offering their child all the gifts of sports, I applaud you.

– Joe Zemaitis

Upcoming *Joe's Rules* books will include Success Stories...
please send me yours...
joe@joesrules.com

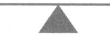

ABOUT THE AUTHOR

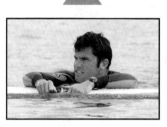

Joe Zemaitis
Athlete • Coach • Teacher

With sixteen years of competitive swimming experience and international accolades as a professional Triathlete, Joe Zemaitis—at age 27—brings a lifetime of experience in competitive sports to his work in coaching and teaching. Joe's coaching philosophy is rooted in the firm belief that every child has a genius—a natural talent that, when recognized and unlocked, paves the pathway to a lifetime of success. Knowing the vast array of critical life skills and lessons learned through sports participation, Joe is a strong proponent of the myriad benefits for every child.

Joe has nine years of coaching experience with swimmers of various ability levels and has built teams of young swimmers who consistently qualify for state, regional, and national competitions. In 2006, he coached and mentored a determined seven-year-old named Braxton Bilbrey who challenged the treacherous waters of the San Francisco Bay to become the youngest swimmer ever to make the 1.4-mile swim from Alcatraz to San Francisco. In that same year, Joe launched Swim Neptune, a year-round competitive USA Swimming

Club that has grown to include five locations across the Phoenix metro area and continues to nurture young swimmers in pursuit of their competitive goals.

In support of childhood drowning prevention and water safety initiatives, Joe created F.A.S.T.— The Foundation for Aquatic Safety and Training. A non-profit organization, based in Phoenix, Arizona, F.A.S.T. was inspired by Braxton Bilbrey's determination in his goal to raise awareness for childhood drowning prevention. The Inaugural Mayoral Race, slated for summer 2007 in Phoenix, will provide yet another forum for awareness campaigns for water safety and training.

As an amateur triathlete, Joe set the 19 and under record at the 1998 Hawaii Ironman Triathlon. Named the 2005 USA Triathlon Professional Rookie of the Year, he set a new course record. In 2003, Joe won the overall Amateur Ironman title in Langkawi, Malaysia. He is a two-time 19 and under National Champion, a seven-time Midwest College Conference Swimming Champion, a three-time Lake Forest College school record holder as well as a six-time Triathalon All-American who represented Team USA at six World Championships. Joe has competed in eleven countries and twenty-seven states and continues to race professionally around the world.

Joe earned a full tuition academic scholarship to Lake Forest College where he graduated in 2002 Summa Cum Laude and Phi Beta Kappa. He was a Rhodes Scholarship finalist and recipient of the Graduating Scholar Athlete Award.

Joe's mission is to shine a national spotlight on the value of sports in every child's life.

He is a sought-after speaker and program facilitator by middle schools, high schools, and parents' organizations across the country for his life skills and success skills seminars. His first book, *Joe's Rules • How Every Parent Can Help Their Child Excel in Life — Through Sports*, was published in 2007 and promises to be the first of a Joe's Rules series dedicated to young people the world over and those who love and support them as they grow to become the leaders and champions of tomorrow.

Joe lives in Phoenix and his parents, John and Helen—as well as siblings John and Amy—continue to play important roles in his life.

RESOURCES AND REFERENCES

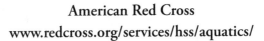

American Red Cross
www.redcross.org/services/hss/aquatics/

Center for Sports Parenting
www.sportsparenting.org

Foundation for Aquatic Safety and Training
www.thefastfoundation.org

President's Council on Physical Fitness and Sports
www.fitness.gov

Swim Neptune
www.swimneptune.com

USA Swimming
www.usaswimming.org

Swim Neptune

Swim Neptune was created to implement my vision for a focused and replicable way to change youth sports for the better. The program focuses on the complete development of a young athlete beginning with the entry-level swimmer and continuing through the collegiate and national athletic arena.

Launched in the fall of 2002, with one location offering practice only three days each week, Swim Neptune has "grown up" with its swimmers. Over the past five years, the Swim Neptune program has grown to meet the huge and growing demand for youth sports programs to become one of the largest in Arizona. Today Swim Neptune, a year-round competitive swimming program, practices seven days a week at five locations in Phoenix, Scottsdale, Glendale, and Chandler. Program options range from two days per week for athletes new to the sport (or who want to swim in addition to other activities in their lives) to an elite track program designed to develop national level athletes.

In the five years I have spent building the team I have been driven by the desire to share my love of the sport of swimming with the next generation of young people and using sport as a venue to show young people the power of goals in all areas of their life. Swim Neptune is the tangible manifestation of that passion and a forum for unlocking the core genius in a young athlete and laying the foundation for the moment of victory.

The activities surrounding the team of Swim Neptune athletes, including the Alcatraz swim and trips to Australia and other international destinations, make it clear to the athletes that there are opportunities with this sport and with Swim Neptune that are unique.

At Swim Neptune, one special and fundamental difference is the coaches. I have worked hard to surround myself with the most accomplished teachers of the sport, coaches who are able to use their own love for and success in the sport to help each individual athlete in the program achieve to the fullest of their individual potential. They share my vision for the future and believe in the Swim Neptune program and its power to positively impact young lives.

– Joe Zemaitis

For more information on Swim Neptune please visit
www.swimneptune.com